MW00396392

THE COMPLETE IDIOT'S GUIDE® TO

The TLC Diet

by Diane A. Welland, MS, RD

ALPHA
A member of Penguin Group (USA) Inc.

To my loving and wonderful husband, Kevin.

ALPHA BOOKS

Published by Penguin Group (USA) Inc.

Penguin Group (USA) Inc., 375 Hudson Street, New York, New York 10014, USA • Penguin Group (Canada), 90 Eglinton Avenue East, Suite 700, Toronto, Ontario M4P 2Y3, Canada (a division of Pearson Penguin Canada Inc.) • Penguin Books Ltd., 80 Strand, London WC2R 0RL, England • Penguin Ireland, 25 St. Stephen's Green, Dublin 2, Ireland (a division of Penguin Books Ltd.) • Penguin Group (Australia), 250 Camberwell Road, Camberwell, Victoria 3124, Australia (a division of Pearson Australia Group Pty. Ltd.) • Penguin Books India Pvt. Ltd., 11 Community Centre, Panchsheel Park, New Delhi—110 017, India • Penguin Group (NZ), 67 Apollo Drive, Rosedale, North Shore, Auckland 1311, New Zealand (a division of Pearson New Zealand Ltd.) • Penguin Books (South Africa) (Pty.) Ltd., 24 Sturdee Avenue, Rosebank, Johannesburg 2196, South Africa • Penguin Books Ltd., Registered Offices: 80 Strand, London WC2R 0RL, England

Copyright © 2013 by Diane A. Welland, MS, RD

All rights reserved. No part of this book may be reproduced, scanned, or distributed in any printed or electronic form without permission. Please do not participate in or encourage piracy of copyrighted materials in violation of the author's rights. Purchase only authorized editions. No patent liability is assumed with respect to the use of the information contained herein. Although every precaution has been taken in the preparation of this book, the publisher and author assume no responsibility for errors or omissions. Neither is any liability assumed for damages resulting from the use of information contained herein. For information, address Alpha Books, 800 East 96th Street, Indianapolis, IN 46240.

THE COMPLETE IDIOT'S GUIDE TO and Design are registered trademarks of Penguin Group (USA) Inc.

International Standard Book Number: 978-1-61564-238-0
Library of Congress Catalog Card Number: 2012944461

15 14 13 8 7 6 5 4 3 2 1

Interpretation of the printing code: The rightmost number of the first series of numbers is the year of the book's printing; the rightmost number of the second series of numbers is the number of the book's printing. For example, a printing code of 13-1 shows that the first printing occurred in 2013.

Printed in the United States of America

Note: This publication contains the opinions and ideas of its author. It is intended to provide helpful and informative material on the subject matter covered. It is sold with the understanding that the author and publisher are not engaged in rendering professional services in the book. If the reader requires personal assistance or advice, a competent professional should be consulted.

The author and publisher specifically disclaim any responsibility for any liability, loss, or risk, personal or otherwise, which is incurred as a consequence, directly or indirectly, of the use and application of any of the contents of this book.

Most Alpha books are available at special quantity discounts for bulk purchases for sales promotions, premiums, fund-raising, or educational use. Special books, or book excerpts, can also be created to fit specific needs. For details, write: Special Markets, Alpha Books, 375 Hudson Street, New York, NY 10014.

Publisher: *Mike Sanders*
Executive Managing Editor: *Billy Fields*
Senior Acquisitions Editor: *Brook Farling*
Development Editor: *Lynn Northrup*
Senior Production Editor: *Kayla Dugger*
Copy Editor: *Krista Hansing Editorial Services, Inc.*
Cover Designer: *Kurt Owens*
Book Designers: *William Thomas, Rebecca Batchelor*
Indexer: *Celia McCoy*
Layout: *Ayanna Lacey*
Proofreader: *John Etchison*

Contents

Appendixes

Introduction

High cholesterol is a serious problem in the United States. According to the Centers for Disease Control and Prevention (CDC), more than 100 million adult Americans, or one out of every three people, has high cholesterol levels (at or above 200 mg/dL). One out of every six Americans has cholesterol levels at 240 mg/dL or above. People with high cholesterol levels (at or above 240 mg/dL) have twice the risk of heart disease than those who have optimal levels (below 200 mg/dL). Furthermore, those who do have high cholesterol are more likely to have other risk factors, like high blood pressure, obesity, and metabolic syndrome.

Fortunately, you can do something about it. Follow the Therapeutic Lifestyle Changes diet, better known as the TLC diet, and you'll not only lower cholesterol levels, but also reduce blood pressure, manage blood sugar levels, and lose weight. Based on years of science and proven to be effective, this government-endorsed diet plan is flexible enough and versatile enough for everyone in your family to enjoy and love. By lowering your cholesterol, you'll reduce your risk of heart disease, the leading cause of death for men and women in America. If you already have heart disease, you can prevent a second event from happening. You'll also feel better, look better, and have more energy throughout the day.

In this book, you'll find everything you need to start living the TLC way, including how and why the TLC diet works, what you should and should not eat, how to clean up your kitchen and navigate grocery shopping, strategies for overcoming bad habits, and tips and techniques to keep you motivated and inspired to stay on track. It's chock-full of practical advice in the form of charts, lists, and savvy substitutions. You'll also find a seven-day weight loss menu plan tailored to 1,200, 1,500, 1,800, or 2,000 calories, and 80 mouthwatering recipes to get you started.

Rated one of the best diets in America for overall good health and sound nutrition by *U.S. News & World Report*, this nutritious diet offers amazing health benefits. Not only will the TLC diet keep your heart running smoothly, but it will also teach you lifestyle habits that will improve your overall health and quality of life. Turn the pages to discover how you can live a long, healthy, and happy life!

How This Book Is Organized

This book is divided into four parts. Each part addresses a different aspect of the TLC diet and includes practical advice for everyday living.

Part 1, Understanding the TLC Diet, explains the why of the diet, including the science behind it and the many health benefits this style of eating has to offer. This part also discusses the basic principles of the diet and goes into detail about fats, carbohydrates, and salt. Here you'll find practical advice on making smart choices for each of those nutrients.

Part 2, Everyday Diet Decisions, talks about what you need to do on a daily level to follow the TLC diet. Here you'll learn how to revamp your kitchen and make room for heart-healthy foods in your pantry, fridge, and freezer; how to navigate the grocery store and make good choices; and what to do about proteins like red meat, fish, cheese, and poultry, the main sources of saturated fat in our diets.

Part 3, Lifestyle Secrets to Success, explains how the TLC program is more than just a diet—it's a lifestyle that promotes regular physical activity and stress management. This part shows you how to plan healthful meals and snacks, using TLC menus as a guideline. It also gives you smart ways to make small dietary changes that make a big difference. Finally, it discusses lifestyle habits that are essential for your success—things like becoming a mindful eater, making good choices when eating out, and keeping a journal. Here you'll find strategies for overcoming bad habits and developing the right mind-set for making a commitment to good health that will last a lifetime.

Part 4, Cooking the TLC Way, introduces you to the wonderful world of healthful and delicious food. In this part, you'll find 80 sensational, heart-healthy recipes that focus on where most people need the most help. I've included chapters on breakfast, the most important meal of the day; beans and grains, two important food groups for controlling cholesterol; flavor boosters to make food pop without salt, sugar, and excess fat; soups, salads, and pizzas; fast and easy favorites; vegan dishes; and, finally, desserts (just because you're on the TLC diet doesn't mean you have to give up sweet treats).

You'll also find two helpful appendixes: a glossary of terms, and additional resources you can find in books, magazines, newsletters, and online.

Extras

In every chapter, you'll find sidebars that feature definitions, tips, warnings, or interesting tidbits you should know about the diet:

DEFINITION

These sidebars highlight definitions of new, sometimes technical words or phrases you may not be familiar with.

HEART-SMART HABITS

These are smart tips and tricks to make following the TLC diet easier and more effective.

GOTCHA!

Here you'll find info on foods or ingredients that you may not realize are high in fat, sugar, salt, or calories. These are foods to go easy on or avoid altogether.

HEALTHFUL LIVING

These sidebars offer trivia and other bet-you-didn't-know information related to the TLC diet.

Acknowledgments

I would like to express my heartfelt thanks to all the people who have helped make this book possible—especially Marilyn Allen, of Allen O'Shea Agency, for offering me such a wonderful opportunity and having the faith in me to do it; all the staff at Alpha Books, especially Brook Farling and Kayla Dugger; development editor Lynn Northrup; Kalle Mace, for her expertise with nutrient analysis, without whose help I would have never gotten done; and everyone who spent time talking to me, including Cynthia Harriman, Julie Miller Jones, Susan Moore, Janet Sass, and all my other RD friends and colleagues who encouraged and supported me throughout this process.

I would also like to thank my gracious friends and family for bearing with me through countless hours of research, not to mention tasting and testing a slew of recipes. This includes my ever-patient and hard-working chef husband, Kevin, and my children, Leslie, Sophia, and Christopher. Without their help and positive motivation, this book would not have been possible.

Special Thanks to the Technical Reviewer

The Complete Idiot's Guide to the TLC Diet was reviewed by an expert who double-checked the accuracy of what you'll learn here, to help us ensure that this book gives you everything you need to know about the TLC diet. Special thanks are extended to Sophia Kamveris.

Sophia Kamveris, MS, RD, LD, is a registered dietitian and licensed nutritionist. Sophia runs a private practice for nutrition and wellness counseling in Boston, Massachusetts, and is a health consultant for the food and beverage industry.

Trademarks

All terms mentioned in this book that are known to be or are suspected of being trademarks or service marks have been appropriately capitalized. Alpha Books and Penguin Group (USA) Inc. cannot attest to the accuracy of this information. Use of a term in this book should not be regarded as affecting the validity of any trademark or service mark.

Medical Disclaimer

The publisher is not responsible for your specific health or medical needs that may require medical supervision. Neither the publisher nor the author is engaged in rendering professional advice or services to the individual reader. The ideas, procedures, and suggestions contained in this book are not intended as a substitute for consulting with your physician. Neither the author nor the publisher is responsible for any adverse reactions to the remedies contained in this book and neither shall be liable for any loss or damage allegedly arising from any information or suggestion in this book.

Understanding the TLC Diet

Part 1

Every year a heart attack strikes more than 1.2 million people, making it the leading killer of both men and women in the United States. But it doesn't have to happen to you. You can reduce your risk of getting a heart attack or prevent another one from occurring simply by changing your dietary and lifestyle habits and following the TLC diet. This healthful diet is designed to lower blood cholesterol levels, a major risk factor for cardiovascular disease, as well as help you control other risk factors, like high blood pressure and obesity. In this part, I discuss exactly what a healthful diet like the TLC diet can do for you and why it's a good way of eating for everyone in your family. I also discuss the nuts and bolts of the diet and explain why monitoring fat and cholesterol is so important for good heart health.

Chapter 1

What Is the TLC Diet?

In This Chapter

- The TLC diet uncovered
- A bounty of health benefits
- What makes it work: ease and flexibility
- A diet for all ages

If you're looking for a sound, nutritious diet that's safe, effective, and easy to follow; reduces your risk of heart attack, stroke, diabetes, and other chronic illnesses; and can help you lose weight, then the Therapeutic Lifestyle Changes diet, better known as the TLC diet, is for you.

Just this year, *U.S. News and World Report* staffers, along with a panel of 22 distinguished health professionals in the field of diet, nutrition, diabetes, and cardiovascular disease, ranked the TLC diet number two in the category of "Best Diet Overall" for these traits: nutrition, safety, ease of use, and protection against diabetes and heart disease. The team, whose goal it was to cut through the clutter and tempting promises and then deliver the facts, evaluated 25 popular diets.

What makes the TLC diet so appealing is more than just its health benefits, which I cover in more depth in this chapter. It's also easy, flexible, and appropriate for everyone from young people, to families with children, to elderly adults. Plus, it's government endorsed: the National Institutes of Health developed this diet plan in May 2001.

So why haven't you heard of it? Probably because, as a government-created diet plan, it didn't have the budget or wherewithal for flashy publicity or big promotional campaigns like other popular consumer diet plans do. Educational efforts originally targeted mainly health professionals and doctors so they could teach patients. But all that's changing as more people become aware of this diet and the many rewards it offers.

Who Developed It and Why?

Back in 1985, the National Heart, Lung, and Blood Institute created the National Cholesterol Education Program (NCEP) and developed two diet guides, Step I and Step II, that were designed to reduce blood cholesterol levels, improve heart health, and lower your chances of having a heart attack. Step I, the less restrictive of the two, was for people who had high cholesterol and two or more risk factors like high blood pressure and diabetes (I'll talk more about risk factors in Chapter 3). It recommended reducing total fat to less than 30 percent, saturated fat to less than 10 percent, and dietary cholesterol to less than 300 milligrams a day. For people who already had heart disease, and to prevent a second heart attack, the Step II diet decreased both saturated fat and cholesterol levels even more, to less than 7 percent total saturated fat and 200 milligrams cholesterol.

Fifteen years later, however, much had changed concerning what we know about heart disease. While keeping total cholesterol—and specifically low-density lipoprotein (LDL)—low is still vital to protecting heart health, we now know that having high blood pressure, diabetes, or metabolic syndrome (more about metabolic syndrome later in this chapter) can also be detrimental to your heart. Furthermore, keeping cholesterol low can help these conditions, too. (I talk more about LDL cholesterol in Chapter 3.)

As a result of this new research, the NCEP introduced the Therapeutic Lifestyle Changes program in May 2001. Stressing a multifaceted approach that emphasizes diet, weight loss, and regular physical activity, the *TLC program* strives to slow the development of coronary heart disease and reduce long-term risk by decreasing LDL and total cholesterol.

DEFINITION

The **TLC program** stands for the Therapeutic Lifestyle Changes program. This comprehensive program, developed by the National Heart, Lung, and Blood Institute of the National Institutes of Health, is aimed at reducing high cholesterol and focuses on diet, physical activity, and weight management.

The earlier you follow the TLC diet, the better. Maintaining a low cholesterol level throughout life, especially in your younger years, offers a greater risk reduction of heart disease and a greater benefit than if you start later in life.

Basic Tenets of TLC

With an eye on prevention, the TLC diet recommends the following:

- **Saturated fat:** Less than 7 percent of total calories
- **Total fat ranges:** From 25 to 35 percent of total calories, with up to 10 percent from polyunsaturated fats and up to 20 percent from monounsaturated fats
- **Dietary cholesterol:** Less than 200 milligrams a day
- **Trans fatty acids:** As low as possible
- **Fiber intake:** 20 to 30 grams of fiber or more a day, with 10 to 25 grams of this fiber coming from soluble fiber
- **Carbohydrates:** 50 to 60 percent of total calories
- **Protein intake:** Range from 10 to 25 percent of total calories, averaging around 15 percent

Health Benefits

While lowering cholesterol is the primary directive of the diet, it's not the only advantage. This therapeutic diet can also improve blood pressure, triglyceride levels, and insulin resistance, and can help you lose weight. Consequently, in addition to benefiting people with heart disease, the TLC diet is recommended for people with diabetes, hypertension, and metabolic syndrome. But don't think that you have to have an illness or special condition to follow this diet. This nutritionally sound, cholesterol-lowering eating plan, based on the USDA 2010 Dietary Guidelines for Americans, is a good diet for anyone and everyone, which is why its popularity and appeal is growing.

Reduces Risk of Heart Disease

Reducing saturated fat in the diet reduces blood cholesterol and, specifically, bad LDL cholesterol, which reduces your risk of *coronary artery disease*, also called coronary heart disease. Coronary artery disease occurs when the arteries leading to your heart narrow, causing decreased blood flow to your heart and damage to the heart muscle. The result is angina, or heart attack.

Coronary artery disease is a type of cardiovascular disease. *Cardiovascular disease* is any condition that affects the structure and function of the heart. Since the TLC diet helps manage factors that contribute to cardiovascular disease, like high blood pressure, diabetes, and metabolic syndrome, it also protects against cardiovascular disease.

DEFINITION

Coronary artery disease occurs when the arteries feeding blood to the heart narrow or close, causing damage to the heart muscle. **Cardiovascular disease** is any condition affecting the function or structure of the heart. Coronary artery disease is a type of cardiovascular disease.

In addition to reducing the foods that can harm your heart, the TLC diet is chock-full of potent foods that help your heart by repairing damaged cells, acting as antioxidants, and reducing inflammation. This ensures that your ticker runs smoothly. Some of the most potent foods include whole grains like oatmeal and flaxseed; veggies like spinach, carrots, and sweet potatoes; fruits like berries; seafood; black beans and kidney beans; nuts; and soy. I talk more about each of these foods in later chapters.

Promotes Weight Loss

Maintaining a healthy weight throughout life not only protects you against heart disease and high cholesterol levels, but also promotes overall good health in general. Being overweight or obese, on the other hand, greatly increases your risk of developing coronary artery disease, high blood cholesterol levels, high blood pressure, and diabetes. Consequently, many people who are overweight or obese have high cholesterol or other conditions that put them at risk for heart disease.

Here's where the TLC eating plan can help. Although the TLC diet isn't considered a weight loss diet, there's a good chance that you'll drop some pounds automatically when you start eating this way. Why? First, you'll be cutting out many processed foods, fatty meats, sugary desserts, and salty snacks that are high in saturated fat and calories. Second, you'll be focusing on foods naturally low in calories, like vegetables, fruits, lean proteins, low-fat dairy, and whole grains. Finally, you'll be moving more by regularly incorporating some type of physical activity into your daily routine.

The good news is that you don't have to lose a lot of weight to reap benefits. All it takes is a few pounds to reduce LDL cholesterol levels, even for people who are overweight or obese.

HEALTHFUL LIVING

In the United States, two out of every three adults are considered overweight or obese. Worse yet is the number of children who are now considered obese—more than 12 million, or one out of every five children. That's more than triple what it was in 1979.

Lowers Blood Pressure

Over time, high blood pressure can lead to heart attack or stroke. Many people with high blood pressure also have high cholesterol. What's considered high? A blood pressure reading of 140 over 90 or greater. The top number represents *systolic* blood pressure, which is the pressure of the heart on arteries when the heart contracts. The bottom number is *diastolic* blood pressure, which measures the pressure of the heart at rest. Normal blood pressure is in the range of 120 over 80.

The TLC diet works to reduce high blood pressure on several fronts. First, it limits salty foods and keeps dietary sodium levels below 2,400 milligrams daily. Second, it emphasizes fruits, vegetables, whole grains, nuts, and low-fat dairy, which are high in potassium, calcium, and magnesium (three nutrients that are known to be blood pressure reducers when sodium is held in check). Finally, this diet helps you lose weight, which also improves blood pressure.

Minimizes Metabolic Syndrome

Metabolic syndrome is actually a cluster of symptoms that when they appear together, greatly increase your risk of heart disease. This is true even when some factors are below heart disease risk. In fact, research shows that metabolic syndrome can raise your chance of developing heart disease and diabetes even if your bad LDL cholesterol is not elevated.

Metabolic syndrome has five features: a big waist, low high-density lipoprotein cholesterol, high blood sugar, high triglycerides, and high blood pressure. If you have at least three of the five features, you have the syndrome.

Abdominal obesity or a large waist and physical inactivity are main signs of the disease. Metabolic syndrome is related to a condition called *insulin resistance*. With insulin resistance, the body cannot properly use the insulin it produces, which can lead to diabetes. Although heredity can play a role in developing the condition, it's more likely that poor diet and lifestyle choices are the real culprits. It comes as no surprise, then, that the cases of metabolic syndrome are increasing. Today about one quarter of all adults in the United States have metabolic syndrome.

Here are specific guidelines for recognizing the five conditions:

- **Big belly:** For women, a waist circumference of 35 inches or more; for men, a waist circumference of 40 inches or more
- **High triglyceride level:** 150 milligrams or higher
- **Low HDL level (high-density lipoprotein, or good cholesterol):** Less than 40 for men; less than 50 for women
- **High blood pressure:** 130/85 mmHg or higher
- **High fasting blood sugar:** 100 mg/dL or higher

If you have or suspect you have metabolic syndrome, never fear. The TLC diet can help you reduce or reverse all of the metabolic syndrome risk factors.

How? When it comes to controlling metabolic syndrome, the two most important factors are losing weight and reducing simple sugars like cakes, cookies, and sweets, and refined carbohydrates such as white pasta, white bread, and white flour. People with metabolic syndrome are particularly sensitive to these foods.

In fact, in some individuals, high-carbohydrate diets ("high" means with 60 percent or more calories coming from carbohydrates) can raise triglyceride levels. By replacing sugary foods and refined carbohydrates with healthier, lower-calorie, high-fiber foods like whole grains, fresh fruits and vegetables, and beans, the TLC diet helps to bring down triglyceride levels and makes it easier to lose weight, particularly around the middle. Alcohol, another well-known cause of high triglycerides, is also something to keep in check on this diet.

GOTCHA!

Everyone knows soft drinks are full of sugar, but did you know energy drinks and sports drinks are no better? Together these three types of beverages make up more than a third of the added sugars we get from our diet, providing us with roughly 8 to 10 teaspoons of added sugar a day.

Manages Diabetes

For people with diabetes, following a TLC diet is especially important because they have a higher risk of heart disease, stroke, and obesity than those without the disease.

For people who don't have the disease but are concerned about getting it, following the TLC plan is also the way to go. That's because the TLC diet restricts foods that are associated with a higher risk of developing diabetes, like sugar-sweetened soft drinks, refined carbohydrates, and certain fatty foods. Instead, the diet emphasizes foods that have a protective effect, like whole grains and fresh fruits and vegetables.

Extra Perks

Part of the reason the TLC diet is gaining so much attention goes beyond the fact that it keeps you healthy and strong and reduces your risk of a number of illnesses. It's also a diet you can live with. Consider that it requires no special foods or diet plans; no tedious, time-consuming preparation methods; and (best of all) no extra expense.

As you begin to eat more plant-based foods and less meat, you will actually save money, as the amount of dollars you spend on food will go down. Furthermore, since food bought in restaurants and food service establishments tends to be high in fat, calories, and sodium, eating out will become more of a special treat than a regular routine. Preparing meals at home costs less than dining out, so this will also save you money. You'll have more income to spend on healthier pursuits, such as joining a gym, playing sports, or buying exercise equipment.

Easy to Follow

The TLC diet emphasizes whole, natural foods that can easily be found at almost any local grocery store, not to mention farmers' markets or specialty stores like Whole Foods. Meal patterns are based on the 2010 Dietary Guidelines MyPlate recommendations (choosemyplate.gov), but modified for a cholesterol-lowering diet. This makes them simple and easy to follow. For this reason, the TLC diet can be easily adapted to suit nearly any lifestyle or eating preference.

In addition to learning about food groups and menu planning, you'll become an expert at reading labels and making smart substitutions. As with any healthful eating plan, you'll be spending more time in the kitchen preparing meals. But in return, you'll be rewarded with high-quality, nutritious foods that will make you feel fit and healthy.

Keep in mind, too, that the TLC diet allows you to include a broad range of foods and meals, so you won't get bored on this diet. In addition to coming up with your own creations and the dozens of recipes included in this book, you can lighten up many high-fat, high-sodium dishes with only a few modifications. This is most true of ethnic cuisines, which tend to focus on vegetables, beans, and whole grains—think Chinese, Mexican, Italian, Indian, Lebanese, and Ethiopian menus—rather than meats.

In fact, the flexibility and versatility of the diet allows you to create fast, flavorful dishes in minutes from any cuisine. See recipes in Part 4 for more ideas.

Live Longer, Live Well

The TLC diet reduces your risk of chronic illness, which, in turn, increases your chances of living a longer, more productive life. But having a good quality of life is more than just being healthy. It also means having an active social life, finding the joy in everyday living, and continuing to grow and learn by being an active member of your community. The TLC diet allows you to be all those things and more by making sure you are performing your best, both physically and mentally.

Who Needs This Diet?

While many people think the TLC diet is only for people who have already had a heart attack or are at high risk of getting one, consuming the right foods to protect your heart is something all people should be doing throughout their life. Consequently, all kinds of people, including young and old, men and women, can benefit from eating this way.

Baby Boomers and Beyond

It makes sense that baby boomers—48 to 66 years of age—and older adults (seniors) would be particularly drawn to the TLC diet. Heart attack risk increases as we age, and not until after the age of 45 for men and 55 for women does age actually becomes a risk factor for heart disease.

As we age, other risk factors creep up on us as well: our blood pressure levels go up, cholesterol levels rise, and the pounds seem to pack on easier. This happens to both men and women. But for women, the estrogen they produce during their reproductive years seems to have a protective effect. Once menopause hits, their chances of getting heart disease dramatically increase; by the age of 65, coronary heart disease becomes much more common for women.

Following the TLC diet is the best way to control these risk factors and significantly reduce your chance of getting a heart attack by 66 years of age, the average age a man has his first heart attack in this country; or 70 years old, the average age a woman has her first heart attack.

Today most first heart attacks are not fatal. And the good news is, cholesterol-lowering therapy like the TLC diet makes a difference, particularly in older adults.

HEALTHFUL LIVING

Men are more likely than women to have excess abdominal weight, which makes them more susceptible to metabolic syndrome and raises their risk of heart disease, particularly in middle age.

Generations X and Y

Many young people assume that because they are in their 20s or 30s, they don't need to worry about heart disease or follow a healthful lifestyle. Nothing could be further from the truth. In fact, some people, young and old, who have heart attacks have no risk factors at all. Following the TLC diet is one of the best things you can do for a "young" heart. Remember, cardiovascular disease—specifically, clogged arteries—doesn't happen overnight. Cardiovascular disease takes years to form and often begins in childhood.

This was brought home in 2007 when researchers looked at the arteries of over 2,800 people who had died between the ages of 15 and 34 years of age. All were victims of accidents, suicides, or homicides and were autopsied shortly after death. The results were striking, particularly for the male subjects (most of them were male). Coronary artery disease was evident as young as 15 years of age and became progressively more apparent over the 20-year age span the study covered.

Poor diet and some extra pounds, however, aren't the only reasons young people are now at risk for heart disease. These Gen Y'ers and X'ers are also more likely to lead stressful, fast-paced lives; get little sleep; and smoke. Smoking at any age does more damage to your heart and your health than any other risk factor.

The TLC diet not only promotes sound nutrition with fresh foods loaded with vitamins, minerals, and fiber, but it also encourages regular physical activity, stress management, and positive lifestyle choices.

Kids and Families

Today one in three children or teens is considered overweight or obese. That's more than triple the rate it was in the 1960s. As a result, many health professionals are seeing more children with heart disease risk factors that were once seen only in adults. Factors like high blood cholesterol, *type 2 diabetes*, and high blood pressure are becoming more prevalent among kids and teens.

DEFINITION

Type 2 diabetes is now the most common type of diabetes in the United States. It occurs when the hormone insulin is inefficient and doesn't do its job, which is to bring fuel in the form of blood sugar to the cells. Once seen only in adults, type 2 diabetes is now being seen in children more and more, thanks to the rise in childhood obesity.

Fortunately, we can do much to reverse this trend. As a parent, your job is to provide your child with the best possible nutrition. Since heart disease and subsequent damage to the heart starts early, if your child has any of these conditions, you need to do something about it. In this case, the TLC diet is a good diet for everyone in your family to follow.

Being a good role model is crucial for the success and the health of your child. In addition to eating well with the TLC diet, encourage family activities that get you moving, limit time spent in front of the TV and computer, and promote positive behavior that's fun and rewarding.

If your child or the rest of your family does not have any health problems, the TLC diet can still be a family affair. There's no need to make separate meals for anyone. The only difference between the TLC diet and other healthful diets is lower intakes of saturated fat and cholesterol. The rest of the diet simply involves good nutrition and sets the stage for teaching your family healthful eating habits that hopefully will stay with them throughout their life.

If something your family wants is not part of your diet plan, the best way to approach this is to offer special "add-on" options. For example, you might offer cheese, nuts, dressings, dried fruit, or a special sauce on the side. Another option is to focus on portion sizes and the proportions of the meal. So instead of taking a larger serving of meat, you would take more vegetables and whole grains and less meat than the rest of the family takes.

Just remember, by sharing your heart-healthy lifestyle with your family, you're also sharing your heart health benefits. What better gift is there?

Minorities

Certain ethnic groups and minority populations are at higher risk of heart disease simply because they are more prone to certain risk factors. For example, African Americans are more likely to have high blood pressure than Caucasians. They are also more likely to have type 2 diabetes, and African American women are two times more likely than white women to be obese, with most of that weight around the abdomen.

Other groups that have a higher prevalence of obesity, diabetes, or other heart disease risk factors include Hispanics, Native Americans, Alaskans, Asian and Pacific Islanders, and South Asians. For these people, following a version of the TLC diet (one using more foods traditional to their culture) is probably a good idea.

Check with Your Doctor

When it comes to a treatment plan for reducing bad LDL cholesterol, always check with your doctor first. Depending on the severity of the case, your doctor could recommend the TLC diet alone or in combination with stronger cholesterol-lowering drugs, like statins.

Nowadays, many doctors routinely check blood cholesterol levels as a matter of course. When and how many times you're checked often depends on how many risk factors you have, if any.

The American Heart Association recommends that everyone over the age of 20 get their cholesterol checked every five years. But if you have any risk factors, your doctor may want to set another schedule, such as annually or every other year. Children are usually screened for cholesterol problems between the ages of 9 and 11.

The Least You Need to Know

- The TLC diet is a cholesterol-lowering diet that limits dietary intake of saturated fats, cholesterol, and sodium.
- In addition to protecting your heart, the TLC diet can help you reduce high blood pressure, lose weight, prevent or manage metabolic syndrome, and control and/or reduce your risk of diabetes.

- Simple and easy to follow, the TLC plan allows you to customize your dietary plan so you can adapt it to suit your lifestyle and eating preferences.
- Both men and women of all ages and ethnicities can benefit by eating the TLC way.
- Be sure to get your blood cholesterol levels routinely screened by a doctor every five years or more.

Chapter 2

TLC Nutrition in a Nutshell

In This Chapter

- Foods to stock up on
- Foods to stay away from
- The value of variety
- Proper portion sizes

The TLC diet is a healthful diet that follows many of the same basic nutrition principles you probably are already familiar with. It emphasizes whole, natural plant foods like fruits, vegetables, whole grains, and beans; includes small amounts of lean meat, fish, and poultry; goes easy on dairy; and focuses on good fats from nuts, seeds, olives, and avocados.

Like all nutritious diets, it stays away from already-prepared items, which tend to be high in fat, sugar, and salt; fried foods and fatty foods; salty snacks like chips; and empty-calorie foods like soft drinks, doughnuts, and pastries.

Instead of concentrating on what you can't have, however, this chapter highlights what you can. It gives you an overview of all the food groups and how they fit into the diet pattern. This way, you can adjust the foods by group to fit your own personal likes and dislikes. Later you'll find more in-depth chapters on specific nutrients like fats, carbohydrates, protein, and sodium to offer more guidance.

Once you start buying and preparing wholesome, natural foods you'll discover a whole new world of foods to explore. Many people are surprised by all the choices available to them. They say variety is the spice of life, but when it comes to the TLC diet, variety is crucial to your success. Not only does it provide you with all the nutrients you need to stay healthy, but it also keeps eating from being boring or repetitive—and you can easily transition it into your own personal lifestyle.

Diet Overview: The Pattern

When it comes to diets, many people want to be told exactly what to eat and when to eat it. These rigid prescriptions never work. Why? Eventually, people get tired of being "told" what to eat and what not to eat. In addition, these diets don't take into account personal likes and dislikes, lifestyle and social factors, habits, and a host of other issues that influence food choices.

Learning a specific pattern of eating is much more flexible and versatile than just following a "diet." Patterns offer an array of options that can accommodate cultural, ethnic, traditional, and personal preferences. Patterns can also be adapted to fit any type of food budget, skills in the kitchen, availability, and time management issues.

The TLC diet pattern is based on the USDA Food Patterns in the 2010 Dietary Guidelines for Americans. It is then adjusted for saturated fat, cholesterol, sodium, and calories. This pattern includes foods from all five major food groups, plus an allowance for fats and oils, solid fats, and added sugars, known as *SoFAS*. Here I've broken the pattern into a few easy principles to live by.

DEFINITION

SoFAS are solid fats and added sugars. Solid fats are solid at room temperature and include butter, margarine, lard, shortening, chicken fat, meat fat, pork fat, and milk fat. Added sugars are sugars added to foods during processing or preparation or at the table.

Focus on Fruits and Vegetables

According to the new MyPlate food guide, fruits and vegetables should make up more than half your plate, and the same holds true for the TLC diet. In fact, filling up half your plate with these good-for-you foods first thing, *before* you even add your protein and starches, is a good habit to get into.

Both fruits and vegetables are loaded with beneficial plant compounds called phytochemicals and antioxidants. Antioxidants fight heart disease by protecting the heart against plaque buildup (you learn more about plaque in Chapter 3). They're also low in fat and calories and high in fiber and potassium, which helps control blood pressure—another perk for helping your heart.

While most of this sounds like common sense, research backs it up. Several large observational studies showed that high fruit and vegetable consumption inversely reduced the risk of heart disease, particularly for middle-aged women. In one study, individuals who ate five or more servings of fruits and vegetables a day had nearly a 20 percent reduction in heart disease risk than those who ate less than three servings a day.

And the more you eat, the better. A 2004 Harvard study comparing highest to lowest intakes found that those who ate eight or more servings of fruits and vegetables a day were 30 percent less likely to have a heart attack or stroke than those who ate only one and a half servings of fruits and vegetables a day.

Although all fruits and vegetables are beneficial, veggies and, specifically, green leafy veggies like spinach, arugula, kale, collard greens, and Swiss chard have an edge. This is because they are such a concentrated source of nutrients like folate, vitamin C, and beta-carotene.

On the TLC diet, aim for 8 to 10 servings of fruits and vegetables a day. Always choose fresh, minimally processed or unprocessed fruits and vegetables that are in season. This gives you both the best taste and the best nutrients (and your selections will be cheaper, too). Be sure to include leafy greens every day, either raw, like in salads (green lettuce counts, too), or cooked.

Up Your Whole Grains and Beans

Whole grains are another mainstay on the TLC diet and are always preferred over white or refined products. Refined grains are foods that have had their nutritious bran or fiber removed during processing, leaving only the starchy part of the grain or kernel. They include white flour, white sugar, white bread, and white rice.

In whole grains, both the bran and the germ are left intact. These two parts of the grain are nutrient powerhouses loaded with fiber and heart-healthy vitamins and minerals like magnesium, selenium, and potassium. Together these nutrients, along with other beneficial plant compounds, like antioxidants, shield the heart from disease. On the TLC diet, at least half of your grain servings should be whole grains.

HEART-SMART HABITS

All it takes is three servings of whole grains a day to protect against heart disease. According to a 2003 study conducted by the University of Minnesota on Atherosclerosis Risk in Communities, three servings of whole grains a day was associated with a 28 percent lower risk of coronary artery disease.

Dried beans are also chock-full of fiber and include similar heart-protecting nutrients. They are particularly high in beneficial soluble fiber. In a large U.S. study of more than 10,000 men and women, eating at least four servings of beans a week was found to lower the risk of heart disease by more than 20 percent. If that's not enough to convince you to up your bean intake, consider that researchers in Japan, Greece, Sweden, and Australia have all linked bean-eaters to greater longevity—so if you want to live longer, eat beans.

Since beans are one of our best sources of plant protein, they are often eaten in lieu of meat. Paired with whole grains, beans make a complete protein, which means they supply all of the body's protein needs. Traditional bean and grain dishes exist in cultures all over the world. For many of these countries, they are a great source of culinary pride—think Louisiana red beans and rice, Indian dahl with whole-wheat naan bread or rice, and Mexican corn tortillas and pinto beans.

On the TLC diet, the best way to up your bean and grain intake is to incorporate two or three vegetarian meals into your diet every week. Once you get used to it, this is easier than you think. Check out Chapter 16 for ideas on how to add more beans and grains to your life.

Lighten Up Your Dairy

Milk and milk products supply the majority of calcium and vitamin D we get in our diet. They are also an excellent source of protein. Unfortunately, these foods are also high in saturated fat and cholesterol. In fact, cheese is the top source of saturated fat in the American diet.

Consequently, the TLC diet limits full-fat dairy products. Instead, you choose low-fat or fat-free versions of nearly all dairy products, including milk, buttermilk, yogurt, sour cream, cottage cheese, cream cheese, and some cheeses.

GOTCHA!

Beware of taking calcium supplements. A new German study looking at 24,000 adults found that those who took calcium supplements were more than twice as likely to have a heart attack than those who didn't take any supplements. Scientists think the fact that supplements provide calcium in one large dose rather than small amounts throughout the day (which is how we get it in food) may be harmful.

Low-fat and fat-free dairy products are a good choice when watching saturated fats, but be aware that many of these products are higher in sodium than their full-fat counterparts. When choosing any low-fat dairy product, be sure to check the sodium content.

Full-fat cheeses are used only when they are high in flavor, such as in a sharp Parmesan, feta, or blue cheese, and in small amounts. For these cheeses, a little goes a long way.

Make Meat a Condiment

Meat, fish, and poultry are three foods you want to keep a close eye on when following the TLC diet. Although they provide high-quality protein and a variety of important vitamins and minerals, like vitamin B_{12}, zinc, and iron, they are also prime sources of saturated fat and cholesterol in the diet.

Furthermore, the amount of fat in these foods can vary considerably, depending on the cut or type of meat, fish, or poultry you choose and how you prepare it. As a general rule, always choose lean cuts of red meat, 93 percent lean ground products, and poultry without the skin (see Chapter 9 for more on this). Seafood is typically low in fat, but here cholesterol is the limiting factor: certain types of seafood are not good choices, particularly shellfish like shrimp, oysters, clams, and mussels.

To keep both saturated fat and cholesterol under control, the TLC diet recommends that most people eat 5 ounces or less of meat, fish, or poultry a day on an average 1,500- to 2,000-calorie diet. However, this number could go up to 6 ounces if calorie levels go higher.

Vegetarians who get their protein from plant sources like legumes, beans, soy, vegetables, and some animal foods like cheese and dairy don't have to worry about these guidelines.

Since most people are accustomed to eating 6 to 8 ounces of these center-of-the-plate entrées *in one meal*, consuming 5 ounces or less for a whole day can be an adjustment. Much of this is a matter of getting into the right frame of mind. Instead of having a large piece of meat surrounded by a few vegetables or grains, you will have a small piece of meat enhanced by an ample amount of vegetables and whole grains.

If you think of meat as a condiment or flavoring ingredient to the grain or vegetables you are serving rather than a center-of-the-plate item, you'll have an easier time planning meals. Here are a few tips to help you get started:

- Slice red meat or chicken in several slices and fan out over the rest of the food.
- Cut meat, chicken, or fish into small pieces and cook with a whole grain or pasta in a pilaf or risotto.

- Make a vegetable stir-fry with a thinly sliced meat, fish, or poultry.
- Feature small amounts of meat, poultry, or fish in soups or stews.
- For a favorite family meal, cut the meat portion in half and double the vegetables and starch.

Watch the Fats

With total fat calories ranging from 25 to 35 percent of total daily calories, the TLC diet is not considered low in fat. It's low in saturated fat, but not total fat. That's okay because it affords more flexibility and better taste than low-fat diets. You'll also be more likely to stick to it through the years.

Most of the fats in the TLC diet are unsaturated, meaning they come from fats that are liquid at room temperature. This includes vegetable oils like canola oil, corn oil, peanut oil, olive oil, soybean oil, and safflower oil, as well as high-fat foods mainly from plants like olives, nuts, seeds, and avocados.

Although unsaturated fats are considered "good" fats, too much of a good thing can still be bad. So while a little is fine, dousing your food in olive oil and deep-frying foods is not a recommended practice. If you do want to up your intake of fats, it's better to look to real foods first rather than liquid fats. In addition to containing "good" fats, these foods provide an array of vitamins, minerals, and fiber.

Fatty fish is one of those foods. High in unsaturated fat, fish like tuna, salmon, and mackerel are popular picks on the TLC diet. The type of fat most common in these fish is called omega-3 fatty acids. *Omega-3 fatty acids* are a kind of polyunsaturated fat that actually protects against heart disease (more about omega-3s in Chapter 4). This is why health professionals recommend eating seafood two to three times per week.

DEFINITION

Omega-3 fatty acids are a kind of polyunsaturated fat that is found in seafood and offers many health benefits, particularly for the heart. It is essential, meaning we need to get it from our diet.

Bad fats are saturated or solid at room temperature. These include butter, lard, fatty grain-based desserts, animal fat, and partially hydrogenated or hydrogenated fats, better known as trans fats. They are found in fatty, grain-based desserts (cookies, cake, and pie); pizza; cheese; and fatty meats. (I talk more about bad fats in Chapter 3.) Bad fats are not only bad for our heart, but also can lead to obesity and a number of other chronic illnesses, like diabetes, cancer, and stroke. These are the fats we want to reduce or even eliminate (as in the case of trans fats).

Eggs over Easy

Eggs are one of the few foods that are low in saturated fat but high in cholesterol. All this fat is located in the yolk, so while egg whites and egg substitutes are not limited on the TLC diet, the whole egg is.

Due to its high cholesterol—new USDA data shows that one egg contains 184 milligrams cholesterol; egg yolks are restricted to only two times per week—this includes baked goods and processed foods. You can have a whole scrambled egg, but you then need to consume no other cholesterol-containing foods for the rest of the day.

Dealing with Drinks

Anytime you're talking about a healthful eating plan, you need to take into account beverages as well as food. That's because a large part of our calorie intake—about 22 percent of total calories, or more than 400 calories—actually comes from what we drink. Most of these calories are in the form of sugary or fatty (creamy) drinks like coolers, milkshakes, or frappuccinos that are not good for our heart or our body.

The best beverages are natural and unsweetened, such as water, nature's own thirst-quencher (plain, sparkling, or carbonated); unsweetened tea and coffee; and fat-free milk. Alcoholic beverages such as wine and beer have a place in this diet, too, and may even offer some health benefits for your heart. I talk more about each of these drinks in Chapter 5, when we look at carbohydrates in more depth.

What You Don't Eat: Salt, Fat, and Sugar

So if those are all the foods you will be eating, what foods will you most likely be giving up? Fatty, salty, and sugary foods with little nutritional value. These foods are called empty calorie foods because they lack nutrients and provide little else but calories. Soft drinks, candy, and pastries are perfect examples of foods that are high in fat, sugar, and calories but offer few vitamins, minerals, or fiber.

Pre-prepared foods (called processed foods) and fast foods also fall into this category. Processed foods are so called because they have been treated or changed in some way to alter their physical, chemical, or sensory properties, usually to enhance palatability or lengthen shelf life. Sometimes they are also referred to as manufactured foods.

Although many foods can be considered processed, the kind of processed foods we are talking about here come out of a box, bag, or can, and contain a large amount of artificial or man-made ingredients. They are usually made from refined grains and, more often than not, are loaded with salt, sugar, fat, and calories. Some examples of processed foods are frozen dinners; macaroni and cheese in a box; canned soups, stews, and chilis; prepared rice, pastas, noodles, and potatoes; and frozen, boxed, or packaged desserts, like cakes, cookies, puddings, and pies.

Since they lack the germ and bran found in whole grains, processed refined foods are generally devoid of fiber, trace minerals, and vitamins that are found in whole-grain, natural, wholesome foods. This means they lack many of the heart-healthy nutrients naturally found in food, too. Processed foods also tend to be high in sodium and low in potassium, both of which foster high blood pressure, a major risk factor for cardiovascular disease.

HEALTHFUL LIVING

Nearly 80 percent of our sodium intake comes from eating processed foods. Much of the time, this salt is hidden, so the food doesn't taste salty.

The TLC diet has no place for processed or convenience foods. Not only do they lack many important nutrients, but the extra fat and calories they provide promote weight gain and poor dietary habits. The high sodium levels also lead to high blood pressure, which taxes the heart. If you want to consume these foods, consider them a special treat to be enjoyed only once or twice a month.

As you adjust to the TLC, you will get better and faster at preparing your own foods at home. After a while, you won't even miss convenience foods. Early on, getting rid of processed foods may be a challenge for people used to eating this type of diet, but it is a necessary step if you want to improve your heart health.

The best advice: clear out all processed foods from your pantry, refrigerator, and freezer. This will make room for all the wonderful foods we've already talked about in this chapter and reduce temptation. It will also force you to start cooking.

Variety Rules

Variety is key to having a healthful diet you can stick with for life. It's also vital for getting all the nutrients you need. To ensure that you're eating a wide array of foods, think about color (in addition to texture and flavor). Include a rainbow of colors on your plate every time you eat, and you can't go wrong. This is important for all food groups, but especially the fruit and vegetable groups.

Consider this rainbow of opportunity:

- **Green:** Contain a wealth of vitamins, minerals, and fiber. *Veggies:* Dark leafy greens like lettuces, kale, chard, and spinach. Cruciferous vegetables like broccoli, brussels sprouts, artichoke, and bok choy, and others like asparagus and peas. *Fruits:* Kiwi, honeydew, green grapes, and limes.
- **Red:** High in vitamin C. *Veggies:* Beets, red cabbage, radishes, and red peppers. *Fruits:* Red apples, cherries, strawberries, raspberries, cranberries, pink grapefruit, and red grapes.
- **Orange/yellow:** Loaded with beta-carotene, a form of vitamin A. *Veggies:* Butternut squash, carrots, sweet potatoes, pumpkin, yellow peppers, and sweet corn. *Fruits:* Cantaloupe, apricots, and most citrus fruits (oranges, pineapple, grapefruit, and more).
- **Blue/purple:** Have powerful antioxidants. *Veggies:* Eggplant, purple tomatoes, carrots, and potatoes. *Fruits:* Blueberries, blackberries, purple grapes, figs, plums, and raisins.
- **White:** Many health-promoting properties—for example, reduces risk of cancer. *Veggies:* Garlic and onion family, cauliflower, potatoes, parsnips, turnips, and mushrooms. *Fruits:* Bananas, white nectarines, and white peaches. Low-fat or fat-free milk and milk products.
- **Brown:** Contains whole grains. Whole grains come in a wide variety of brown colors and include oatmeal, barley, quinoa, brown rice, whole-wheat pasta, kamut, faro, teff, kashi, and millet. Legumes or dried beans, lentils, and chickpeas all come in a wide variety of colors, shapes, and sizes, including red, blue, black, yellow, green, brown, and mottled.

Proper Portions

Since 1977, Americans have upped their caloric intake by some 500 calories, from eating about 1,800 calories a day to averaging some 2,300 calories per day by 2003. That would be okay if Americans were burning more calories exercising or being active, but over this time period, we have not increased the amount of physical activity we typically engage in. In fact, we're actually doing less, largely thanks to the advent of the computer.

Excess energy is likely stored as fat. Over the long term, it can build up and lead to weight gain. As a result, we now have generations of overweight adults, a problem with childhood obesity, and a dramatic rise in chronic illnesses related to poor diet, such as heart disease, cancer, and diabetes.

What is causing us to eat so much more than we used to? Although this is a complex answer influenced by individual physical, emotional, and environmental factors, we know that a big part of the problem has to do with how much food is around. Studies on human behavior show many triggers for overeating, but one major cue is simply having more food put in front of us. This is what has exactly happened here in the United States.

Over the last 30 years, *portion sizes* at restaurants have ballooned drastically, increasing in size by several hundred calories or more. Take, for example, a typical muffin, which weighed $1\frac{1}{2}$ ounces and now clocks in at 4 ounces. Likewise, pizza has gone from a slice of about 5 ounces to a personal pie at 13 ounces. Other big gainers since 1980 include cookies (seven times larger), pasta (five times larger), steaks (doubled), and drinks (two to three times bigger).

Unfortunately, we have gotten so used to these bigger portion sizes that now we also serve them at home. Bigger portions mean bigger people. Plus, portion sizes are not the same as *serving sizes.* Portion sizes are based on a variety of factors, including value, expectations, and hunger; serving sizes are a standard measure of a typical amount. The TLC diet is based on serving sizes.

DEFINITION

Portion size is the amount of food that is customarily served in a home or restaurant setting. **Serving size** is the amount of a single serving of food, based on a typical portion and determined by the USDA. Serving sizes vary, depending on the type of food.

What Counts as a Serving?

Now that you're on the TLC diet, it is important for you to understand what a serving size is. Serving sizes vary, depending on the kind of food you are eating. However, they follow a specific pattern, which makes it easier to remember. For more information on serving sizes, go to choosemyplate.gov and look at the individual food groups.

Most fruits and vegetables:

$\frac{1}{2}$ cup vegetable = 1 serving

$\frac{1}{2}$ cup fresh fruit = 1 serving

1 cup berries or melon = 1 serving

1 medium piece of fruit = 1 serving (banana, apple, orange, peach, and so on)

1 medium baked potato = 1 serving

1 cup leafy green (spinach or lettuce) = 1 serving

$\frac{1}{4}$ cup dried fruit = 1 serving

6 oz. 100 percent fruit juice = 1 serving

Whole grains:

1 serving from the grains group is equivalent to 1 ounce of grain

1 cup cereal = 1 serving

1 slice of bread = 1 serving (sandwich is 2 servings or 2 ounces)

$\frac{1}{2}$ cup cooked brown rice, whole-wheat pasta, or potato = 1 serving

$\frac{1}{2}$ cup cooked oatmeal = 1 serving

3 cups popcorn = 1 serving

Dairy group:

1 cup (8 ounces) fat-free or 1 percent milk = 1 serving

1 cup nonfat or low-fat yogurt = 1 serving

$1\frac{1}{2}$ ounces cheese = 2 slices of cheese ($\frac{3}{4}$ ounce each) = 1 serving

$\frac{1}{2}$ cup low-fat ice cream = 1 serving

Protein group:

3 ounces meat, fish, or poultry = 3 ounces protein (generally, this is a portion size)

$\frac{1}{2}$ cup cooked dried beans = 2 ounces protein

1 egg = 1 ounce protein

1 tablespoon peanut butter = 1 ounce protein

1 ounce nuts (for example, 25 almonds, or 7 whole or 14 halves walnuts) = 2 ounces protein (for more on nut nutrition, see lancaster.unl.edu/food/ftmar04.htm)

How Do You Measure Up?

How do you know whether the portion on your plate is a serving size? Measure it. Though it's not possible to do when dining out, you can ask the waitstaff what the portion size is that is being served. At home you can—and should—start measuring food amounts with a scale and household measures. This is vital to the success of your diet and helps you in two ways. First, it gets you used to seeing what an appropriate serving size is. Second, it ensures that you are not overeating. People also find it helpful to compare amounts to common items they are familiar with. For example:

1 cup is about the size of a baseball.

3 ounces of meat or poultry is about the size of a deck of cards or a checkbook.

3 ounces of grilled fish is about the size of a checkbook.

$1\frac{1}{2}$ ounces of cheese is equivalent to four stacked die.

2 tablespoons of peanut butter is the size of a Ping Pong ball.

1 teaspoon is the size of the tip of a thumb.

As you become more familiar with serving sizes and practice this technique at home, you will eventually be able to simply eyeball a food and know how much an amount is and how it will fit into your diet. This takes less time than you think; within a week or so, you will be a pro at identifying amounts.

HEALTHFUL LIVING

Research shows that most people underestimate the calories they take in on average by about 30 percent. The larger the meal, the higher the error.

Like anything new, eating the TLC diet way takes some getting used to and requires a bit more work at the start. But in no time, many of the changes you implement now will become like second nature. The key is developing a diet plan that works for you and your family over the long term.

The Least You Need to Know

- On the TLC diet, three quarters of your plate should consist of vegetables, fruits, and whole grains.
- Meat, poultry, and fish should be condiments to enhance the rest of the meal.
- To ensure that you're getting all the nutrients and fiber you need, include an array of colorful foods on every plate.
- Avoid processed and prepared foods, which can be high in fat, calories, sugar, and sodium.
- Be aware of portion sizes so you don't overeat.

Chapter 3

All About Cholesterol

In This Chapter

- Understanding cholesterol and why we need it
- How much is too much?
- Recognizing foods that raise cholesterol
- Knowing what you can and can't do about it

As you know, the TLC diet is a healthful diet designed to reduce your risk of getting heart disease or to decrease the chances of having another heart attack or other heart problems. The focus is primarily on lowering blood cholesterol levels. So what's so bad about cholesterol? In this chapter, I tell you everything you need to know about this often misunderstood fat—where it comes from, what it does in the body, why we need it, and why too much of it can lead to heart disease and increased risk of heart attack.

Many people see cholesterol as a dietary villain and think that if they cut cholesterol out of their diet, their health will automatically improve. That's just not true. Dietary cholesterol is actually the least of our worries when it comes to improving blood cholesterol levels. Trans fats and saturated fats have an even greater impact on blood cholesterol levels and are much harder to control in the diet than cholesterol. Furthermore, carbohydrates, especially in the form of simple sugars, can also negatively affect cholesterol. Although I touch on carbohydrates in this chapter, I talk more about it in Chapter 5.

You can take plenty of actions to reduce blood cholesterol levels, but some things you can't change. Understanding these risk factors will help you better manage your health and your blood cholesterol levels. I talk about each one in the pages that follow.

Cholesterol in Your Body

Cholesterol is a waxy, fatlike substance that is part of a group of compounds call sterols. Sterols are a type of fat or lipid found in the body. Cholesterol is the most famous of the sterols and also one of the most important. In fact, it is essential to life and is found in every cell in your body; it makes up the structure of the cell wall and allows fat-soluble substances to move back and forth freely.

In addition, cholesterol is required to make sex hormones like estrogen and testosterone; the active form of vitamin D; and bile, a necessary component of fat digestion. Even if you ate no cholesterol at all, your body would produce enough cholesterol (as much as 1,000 milligrams) to keep you running smoothly, thanks primarily to the liver, the organ responsible for the management and production of cholesterol.

To get the cholesterol where it's needed, the liver wraps it up in tiny protein-covered packages called lipoproteins. Those lipoproteins are then transported in the blood. The two most important lipoproteins when discussing heart disease are *LDL* and *HDL*. I talk about each of these individually, as well as another fat compound called *triglycerides*.

DEFINITION

LDL, or low-density lipoprotein, refers to tiny particles composed mainly of cholesterol that travel in the blood. **HDL,** or high-density lipoprotein, consists of bigger particles composed mainly of protein that remove cholesterol from the blood. **Triglycerides** are fats that come directly from the food we eat.

In a healthy individual who eats a healthful diet, the liver naturally adjusts the amount of cholesterol it produces to match the amount eaten. When you eat a poor diet or your liver is not working properly, too much cholesterol can build up in the bloodstream, leading to heart disease.

LDL: The Bad Cholesterol

LDL, or low-density lipoproteins, refer to tiny particles composed primarily of cholesterol and a few other fats that travel through the bloodstream, releasing their contents to the cells that need it throughout the body. The liver makes the cholesterol found in LDL.

When too much LDL circulates in the bloodstream, the excess sticks on the artery walls and forms a thick, hard substance called *plaque*. Over time, plaque can build up, causing the blood vessels to narrow and making them less flexible. This condition is called atherosclerosis, or hardening of the arteries.

Plaque buildup on coronary arteries can block nutrient- and oxygen-rich blood from going to the heart. If the artery is partially blocked, it can lead to chest pain or angina. If the artery is completely blocked and no blood is getting through, heart tissue will die, resulting in a heart attack.

Because LDL promotes plaque formation and inflammation, it is considered "bad" cholesterol. High levels of LDL in your blood are considered a major risk factor, significantly increasing your risk of heart disease.

HEALTHFUL LIVING

Most people get about one third of their cholesterol from the food they eat; the liver manufactures the rest. Of what we eat, only about 40 to 60 percent is absorbed.

HDL: The Good Cholesterol

HDL, or high-density lipoprotein, is the heaviest and most dense of the lipoproteins, containing high levels of protein and little fat. HDL is made in the liver and designed to roam the bloodstream picking up cholesterol from dying cells and other sources and bringing it back to the liver to be removed from the body.

Another beneficial function of HDL is that it prevents the oxidation of LDL and reduces inflammation. Oxidized LDL is stickier than nonoxidized LDL and more likely to attach to artery walls, forming plaque.

Because they get rid of excess cholesterol and protect against plaque, HDL is known as "good" cholesterol. High levels are desirable and can even negate the effects of having high LDL. Thus, high HDL can significantly reduce your risk of heart disease.

Triglyceride Levels

Triglycerides are yet another type of fat circulating in the bloodstream. Although not considered a cholesterol or a sterol, high triglyceride levels can be particularly harmful to your heart, potentially increasing your risk of heart disease or stroke by as much as four times. It is especially dangerous when paired with low HDL and high LDL.

Triglyceride levels are produced from the fat we eat, so when the fat content in our diet is high, chances are, our triglyceride levels will be, too. In some people, simple carbohydrates and alcohol raise blood triglyceride levels, too.

Since triglycerides are also the form of fat that is stored as fat cells, eating a high-fat or high-sugar diet not only raises blood triglyceride levels, but also causes you to put on weight.

Although high triglyceride levels are usually paired with other risk factors, such as being overweight and having metabolic syndrome or diabetes, more research is showing that high triglycerides alone may be an independent risk factor for heart disease.

HEART-SMART HABITS

Excess calories from any nutrient—fat, carbohydrate, protein, or alcohol—is converted to triglycerides and stored as fat in the body. This is why it is important not to overeat any food on a regular basis.

Cholesterol in Your Diet

In our diet, cholesterol is found only in animals and animal products. Cholesterol-containing foods include red meat, fish, poultry, eggs, milk, and milk products (like cheese, butter, yogurt, and cream).

Some plants do contain fats called sterols, but these are in the form of plant compounds. Although they are similar in structure to cholesterol, they do not raise cholesterol in the blood. In fact, studies show that they actually have the opposite effect and lower total cholesterol levels.

For years, we thought dietary cholesterol was the primary culprit behind high cholesterol levels, driving heart disease in this country. Years of scientific research now show that saturated fats and trans fats are far worse than dietary cholesterol when it comes to raising blood cholesterol levels in the body—especially bad LDL cholesterol.

Nevertheless, reducing high-cholesterol foods is a good idea and a vital part of the TLC diet. That's because most high-cholesterol foods are also high in saturated fat, with two exceptions. Both eggs and shellfish are high in cholesterol but low in saturated fat, meaning they can be included in the TLC diet in small amounts. Current dietary recommendations are 300 milligrams of dietary cholesterol per day for healthy adults and 200 milligrams of dietary cholesterol per day for those who already have heart disease or are at high risk.

Sans the Saturated Fat

Saturated fats are solid at room temperature. They come from both animals and plants and are most familiar to us in the form of fat in red meat like beef, pork, or lamb; poultry, like chicken and turkey (mainly under the skin and in pockets); lard; and dairy foods like butter, cheese, whole milk, and whole-milk products. In the plant kingdom, saturated fats are found in coconut oil, palm oil, palm kernel oil, and cocoa butter.

When it comes to raising blood cholesterol levels, saturated fats are bad news. They significantly increase LDL levels and total cholesterol levels and promote blood clotting. Eating a diet high in saturated fat is thus a major risk factor for developing high cholesterol and, subsequently, heart disease. A diet high in saturated fat also increases your risk of obesity and diabetes, two other factors that can bump up your chance of having a heart attack.

Of all the foods in your diet, saturated fats are the most detrimental to your heart, partly because of the damage they do to the arteries (via cholesterol) and partly because of the large amounts eaten in a typical diet.

In the United States, the top two sources of saturated fat in the diet are cheese and pizza. These are followed by a slew of dairy and meat products. Cutting back on saturated fats will help your heart and your health, but only if you don't replace these foods with refined carbohydrates and simple sugars. Upping your intake of refined carbohydrates like pastas and bread and simple sugars like soft drinks not only adds more calories, making you more likely to gain weight, but, as mentioned earlier, can also raise LDL and triglycerides, hurting your heart. Instead, replace saturated fats with healthier unsaturated fats, like polyunsaturated and monounsaturated fats.

The 2010 Dietary Guidelines recommend making saturated fat no more than 10 percent of your total calories. The TLC diet takes this one step further, limiting saturated fat to less than 7 percent of total calories. How much is that?

Total Calorie Levels per Day	Saturated Fat in Grams Allowed per Day*
1,200	8
1,500	10
1,800	12
2,000	13
2,200	15
2,500	17

**Equals about 6 percent of total calories*

The Trouble with Trans Fats

Trans fats, or trans fatty acids, is a type of man-made fat produced by a process called *hydrogenation.* During hydrogenation, single hydrogens bombard an unsaturated fat, effectively making it saturated. This produces a product that goes from a liquid to a solid or semi-solid at room temperature (as with margarine). It also results in a creamy texture and a longer shelf life. Since hydrogenated fats are cheap and highly stable, many are also used for frying in food service operations. On labels, trans fats are known as "partially hydrogenated fats." While these traits may be desirable for food manufacturers and restaurants, they aren't so good for us humans.

DEFINITION

Hydrogenation is a man-made process in which unsaturated fats are bombarded with hydrogens and transformed into trans fats. Trans fats raise cholesterol and increase the risk of heart disease. Hydrogenation alters texture and increases the shelf life of food products.

When it comes to heart disease, man-made trans fats are even more dangerous than saturated fats. That's because, in addition to raising LDL cholesterol, trans fats lower HDL cholesterol. Luckily, the amount of trans fats in our diet has significantly dropped over the last few years, thanks to new labeling laws that require listing trans fats on the nutrition facts panel and campaigns to prompt local legislators to force whole cities to become trans fat free.

Today trans fat products make up only a small portion of our diet (about 2.5 percent of total calories), but for most of us, even that small amount is too much. In the TLC diet, trans fats should be kept very low, at 1 percent of the total calories or about 2 grams, and these should be in the form of trans fats found only in nature—small amounts are found in meat and dairy foods. This form of trans fat does not affect cholesterol the way the man-made type does, so it is not considered harmful.

Work to eliminate man-made trans fats. This really isn't as hard as you might think, especially since there are many trans-fat-free products on the market. Like simple sugars and refined carbohydrates, trans fats are found only in processed foods. If you stay away from them, you're sure to stay away from trans fats. Be aware that many products labeled as 0 trans fats could contain small amounts, .5 gram per serving, that can add up if you eat more than one serving.

Monounsaturated and Polyunsaturated Fats

Monounsaturated fats and polyunsaturated fats are considered good fats because they do not raise blood cholesterol—in some cases, they may even have a protective effect against heart disease. These fats are unsaturated, which means they are liquid at room temperature and are most often in the form of vegetable oils. However, nuts, seeds, olives, avocados, and fatty fish like salmon are also classified as unsaturated fats.

When it comes to the TLC diet, monounsaturated fats like olive, peanut, and canola oil and polyunsaturated fats like corn oil, salad oil, and soybean oil should make up the bulk of your fats. Beware, however, of using too much. Even with "good" fats, calories can rack up fast, negating many of their positive effects.

Luckily, you have plenty of room to play with. On the TLC diet, total fat intake ranges from 25 to 35 percent, allowing for more flexibility on menus and a sprinkling of heart-healthy nuts (when appropriate).

Why so high? Despite popular opinion and years of major health organizations telling us to reduce dietary fat, the tide has turned. Mounting evidence shows that the *type* of fat you eat is more important than the amount, and diets restricting fat don't work. In fact, keeping fat levels on the moderate to high side is good for your heart.

Over the last 10 years or so, several large studies, including the Women's Health Initiative and the Nurses' Health Study, have shown no difference in health outcomes like heart disease and weight gain in women following a normal-fat diet versus a low-fat one. This supports the notion that low-fat diets do not protect against heart disease and may even potentially increase risk.

For this reason, health and nutrition authorities have lightened up their message. While eating too much fat is still something to be wary of, adding some healthful extra fats in the form of nuts or seeds is a good thing. Not only can it help your heart, but it also has extra benefits, like making food taste better, keeping you full and satisfied longer so you won't feel hungry or deprived between meals, and making you more likely to stick to the diet for life.

Is Your Number Up?

Now that you know the types of fats your doctor will be looking at when taking your blood lipid profile, it's time to look at the numbers.

If you already have heart disease or other risk factors, you may want your LDL to come down even lower than normal. At the same time, you want your HDL to go up. I've given you some guidelines for that here. All are in mg/dL.

Total cholesterol falls into three categories:

- **Good:** Your numbers are within the normal range, and you can keep doing what you're doing.
- **Keep an Eye On:** You are not considered high risk yet, but you're heading in that direction; you're borderline high.
- **High Risk:** You are at risk for heart disease and/or a heart attack, and you need to bring your numbers down (or up if it's for HDL). This may require medication, depending on what your doctor says.

	Good	Keep an Eye On	High Risk
Total cholesterol	<200	200–239	>240

HDL is categorized as either good or high risk:

- **Good:** You are in good standing; your numbers are high and you should keep up the good work.
- **High Risk:** You are at risk for heart disease; your numbers are too low. You need to work on bringing them up.

	Good	High Risk
HDL	>60	<40

For LDL and triglycerides, there are two additional categories:

- **Pretty Close:** You are near the optimal level but aren't quite there—it's something to strive for.
- **Very High:** You may require immediate medical attention (such as prescription drugs) to bring the numbers down.

	Good	Pretty Close	Keep an Eye On	High Risk	Very High
LDL	<100	100–129	130–159	160–180	>190
Triglycerides	<100	100–149	150–199	200–499	>500

Risk Factors You Can Change

The good news is, if you've decided to follow the TLC diet, you're taking charge of your health. You're motivated enough to make some changes, and you're ready to reduce your risk of heart disease. The bad news is, if you've decided to follow the TLC diet, you probably already have at least one major risk factor for developing heart disease in the future. You may have already been diagnosed with heart disease or even had a heart attack.

HEALTHFUL LIVING

Risk factors are conditions or behaviors that increase your risk of heart disease. Often these risk factors cluster together, so instead of having just one risk factor, most people have two or three or four.

Never fear, however—you can still improve your health. That's because you can change, improve, or even eliminate many risk factors. I've already talked about high blood cholesterol levels (high LDL and low HDL) and high triglycerides as major risk factors for developing heart disease. This is one of the major risk factors for heart disease and the one you most want under control.

Some of the risk factors discussed here have independent effects; others work by raising bad LDL cholesterol, lowering good HDL, increasing blood pressure, and causing inflammation and poor health in general. Here is a rundown of risks you can change and what you can do to turn them around.

Poor Diet

Poor diets high in saturated fat, trans fats, cholesterol, sodium, and sugar increase risk of heart disease by raising total blood cholesterol, LDL, and triglycerides. They can also cause a host of other ailments not good for your heart, including high blood pressure, obesity, and high blood glucose levels.

Risk reducer: Practice good nutrition. Follow a healthful diet like the TLC diet, limiting saturated fat, trans fats, and cholesterol. Cut out empty calories in the form of simple sugars and salt, and increase your intake of high-fiber whole grains, legumes, fruits, and vegetables.

Although the results of dietary changes vary depending on the individual, if you stick to the TLC diet, you may be able to lower bad cholesterol (LDL) 10 to 20 percent after only six weeks. Add in other lifestyle factors, like exercising and losing weight, and you can drop even lower—another 5 to 8 percent.

Physical Inactivity

No one has to tell you that a sedentary lifestyle that revolves around sitting all day is bad, but it is particularly bad for your heart. A 2011 study published in *European Heart Journal* found that sitting for long periods of time, even for people who did a lot of exercise otherwise, was associated with worse indicators of cardio-metabolic function and inflammation, such as larger waist circumferences, lower levels of HDL ("good") cholesterol, and higher levels of triglycerides.

Risk reducer: Get moving! Regular moderate to vigorous physical activity is a must on the TLC diet. Not only will it keep you healthy, fit, and trim, but it also can improve blood pressure and levels of blood cholesterol, triglycerides, and insulin. In addition, staying active offers many mental advantages, by keeping your brain sharp, reducing depression, and helping you sleep better. According to the American Heart Association, you should aim for 30 minutes a day at least five days a week—and more, if you can.

Just remember, doing something is always better than doing nothing. So if you think you don't have time, exercising as little as 10 minutes at a time several times a day may still offer some health benefits. This is also good for sedentary people who should start out slow. Studies show that people who have achieved even a moderate level of fitness are much less likely to die early than those with a low fitness level.

What happens if you sit for long periods of time at work? Take a break often. Get up and walk around every 20 minutes or so. The break will not only keep you healthy, but also can clear your mind and help you work better.

Obesity or Overweight

Being overweight puts you at risk for a host of problems, including high cholesterol, high blood pressure, and insulin resistance, a potential precursor of type 2 diabetes. It also often goes hand in hand with a sedentary lifestyle and poor diet.

Extra weight around the abdominal area, in particular, is especially dangerous for heart disease and other illnesses. To see if your belly is too big, measure your waist circumference. If you're a woman, this means a waist of over 35 inches; if you're a man, it's over 40 inches.

Risk reducer: Lose weight. Gradual weight loss of 1 to 2 pounds a week is the key to success. To do this, follow these three simple steps: switch to a healthful TLC diet, reduce caloric levels by 500 calories a day, and increase physical activity by exercising regularly. For more tips on shedding pounds on the TLC diet, see Chapter 10.

GOTCHA!

You don't have to be overweight to have high cholesterol. In fact, thin people can also be at risk. Often people who don't gain weight are less aware of the amounts of saturated fats and trans fats they eat. Consequently, their diet can be worse.

Smoking

Smokers have a two to four times greater risk of developing heart disease than nonsmokers. Even if you don't smoke, regular exposure to secondhand smoke can increase your risk of heart disease. How? Smoking boosts a person's genetic link to cardiovascular disease by narrowing arteries, elevating blood pressure, and thickening the blood. It also negates the natural protective effect premenopausal women have over men (see "Gender," later in the chapter). Furthermore, women who take oral contraceptives and smoke have an even greater risk of heart disease.

Risk reducer: Pick a date that you will quit smoking and tell all your friends. This way you are setting up a support network. Plan for challenges and don't be discouraged if you don't succeed the first time. It may take several tries to finally give up smoking. When you do, however, you'll begin to feel the effects (and feel better) almost immediately, as your body will begin to heal the moment you stop.

Chronic Stress

Chronic stress promotes heart disease in two ways. First, it can trigger the body to produce a "fight or flight" stress response, which constricts coronary arteries and promotes blood clots. Second, it causes many stressed-out people to overeat or eat poorly, overlook exercise, and smoke.

Risk reducer: Reduce stress. Stress-management techniques range from yoga and meditation to vigorous exercise. Try some different options and then pick the one that's right for you. Remember, eating right, getting the right amount of sleep, and exercising can go a long way in improving how you handle stress.

Diabetes

Adults with diabetes are two to four times more likely to have heart disease or a stroke than adults without diabetes, and about 75 percent of people with diabetes die of some form of cardiovascular disease. That's because people with diabetes are more likely to suffer from high blood pressure, blood lipid level problems, and obesity, a result of long-term damage from elevated blood sugar levels.

Risk reducer: Follow a healthful lifestyle and diet, exercise regularly, and keep diabetes under control. While you can't get rid of diabetes, you can alleviate much of the risk associated with heart disease by keeping blood sugar levels under control, following a healthful diet, exercising regularly, maintaining a healthy weight, keeping blood pressure low, keeping cholesterol and triglyceride levels in line, and not smoking.

People who don't have diabetes but are at high risk for getting it (via genetics or a strong family history) should follow the same advice. Follow the TLC diet, exercise regularly, keep your weight down, and try to reduce stress.

High Blood Pressure

High blood pressure increases the heart's workload, causing damage to the heart muscle by making it thicker and stiffer. High blood pressure also increases your risk of stroke, heart attack, kidney failure, and congestive heart failure. Combined with other risk factors, like obesity, smoking, high blood cholesterol levels, and diabetes, the risk of heart attack or stroke increases greatly. People with diabetes and high blood pressure have double the risk of developing heart disease than people without those conditions.

Risk reducer: Reduce high blood pressure. The best way to do this is to eat the TLC way, exercise regularly, reduce stress, limit alcohol intake, and maintain a healthy weight.

Metabolic Syndrome

As I discussed in Chapter 1, metabolic syndrome is actually a cluster of symptoms that include three or more of the following: large waist circumference, high triglycerides, low HDL, high blood glucose, high LDL, and high blood pressure.

Risk reducer: Reverse or reduce metabolic syndrome symptoms. You can do this by becoming physically active, achieving a healthy weight, and following the TLC diet.

Risks You Can't Change

Knowing the risk factors you can't change makes it even more important to change the risks that you can. Not until my husband had a heart attack at 53, with only one risk factor, and showed a poor total cholesterol profile did we find out that he had a strong history of heart disease in his family. Genetics is not something you can change, but being aware of this factor would have made us more diligent in watching his diet and improving his blood cholesterol numbers.

Age

No one can turn back the hands of time, but it is good to be aware that cardiovascular disease increases as we age. Approximately four out of five people who die of heart disease are over age 65.

Gender

Men have a greater chance of having a heart attack than women—and having one at an earlier age. Even after menopause, when women's rate of heart disease goes up, their risk is still not as high as men's. The good news is, this means men are more likely to recognize heart disease risk and symptoms if they occur and can seek immediate help.

Heredity

Family history can play a strong role in determining whether you are susceptible to heart disease. If someone in your immediate family died of heart disease at a young age, it's important to realize that you are now at high risk. To prevent this from happening to you, controlling other risk factors like diet, exercise, and high blood pressure becomes even more important.

Race can affect heart disease risk, too. For example, heart disease is more common in Caucasians than it is in African Americans. Rates of cardiovascular disease are also higher among Hispanic/Latino, Native American, and native Hawaiian groups. This is partly because these groups also have high levels of diabetes and obesity.

Your Genes

You may not have any of the previous risk factors, but your liver may not be working properly, leading to high blood cholesterol and high triglyceride levels. This is most obvious when children have high blood cholesterol levels and no other risk factors. Genetic hypercholesterimia (high total cholesterol and LDL) is the most common type of genetic disorder that can increase your risk of heart disease. And although you can't change your genes, with lifestyle changes, good nutrition (like following the TLC diet), and possibly medication, you can keep these risk factors at bay.

The Least You Need to Know

- Cholesterol is an essential compound that the body produces, but excess cholesterol can build up in your bloodstream and cause hardening of the arteries and heart attack.
- To reduce your risk of heart disease, you want total cholesterol and LDL cholesterol low, HDL cholesterol high, and triglyceride levels low.
- The best way to protect yourself from heart disease is to exercise regularly, reduce stress, keep weight in check, and follow the TLC diet.
- When it comes to cardiovascular disease, you can change only some risk factors, but you will still benefit from eating a TLC diet.

In the Know About Fats

Chapter 4

In This Chapter

- The best of the bunch: avocados, olives, nuts, and seeds
- Finding ways to fit in fish
- Avoiding fats that harm your heart
- Why not all saturated fats are bad

In the nutrition world, fats have always gotten a bad rap. They're blamed for nearly all of our ever-growing health problems, and for decades, health professionals have urged people to cut the total fat in their diet. It's true that eating too much of this concentrated source of calories can make you fat, increase your risk of chronic illness, and crowd out other more nutritious foods. But fat is vital to good health. It's necessary for immune function, digestion, sex hormones, healthy skin and hair, and proper brain function. So it's not surprising to find that the low-fat diets once touted have not panned out. New research proves that it's not the amount of fat that we eat—it's the type of fat.

When it comes to taking care of your heart and your health, you want to steer clear of saturated fats and trans fats. These are the worst kind of fats for you, but not all of them are created equal. Recent research shows that some types of saturated fatty acids may not be that bad and may even have some redeeming qualities; you'll see this later when I discuss butter, chocolate, and coconut oil.

What's most important is to replace the bad fats, like saturated fat, not with carbohydrates or sugars, but with healthy fats, like polyunsaturated and monounsaturated fats. I show you how in this chapter. These fats not only take the place of harmful fats in your diet, but they also have protective qualities of their own and can keep your heart running smoothly.

With as much as 35 percent of calories coming from fat (or roughly 77 grams on a 2,000-calorie diet), the TLC diet isn't considered a low-fat plan. Instead, it's a healthful, heart-smart diet. By replacing much of the saturated fat with healthier polyunsaturated and monounsaturated fats, this diet benefits not just your heart—it's also good for your stomach (so you feel full longer), your taste buds, and your mind. You'll have an easier time sticking to this plan for life.

The only time fat and calories are a concern is when you're trying to lose weight. I cover that in Chapter 10. For now, don't be afraid to have some fat in your diet—just make sure it's the good kind.

Fats You Need More Of

Fats usually come in two forms: solid and liquid. The solid fats are solid at room temperature and high in saturated fats and trans fats. The liquid ones are liquid at room temperature and high in unsaturated fats. As a general rule, you want to pass up solid fats and go for liquid fats.

Certain foods are also high in fat. In the plant kingdom, high-fat foods contain mostly good fats, like monounsaturated fats and polyunsaturated fats, which decrease cholesterol levels and inflammation and help regulate heart rhythm. They have the added bonus of vitamins, minerals, fiber, and phytochemicals. These fats are found in avocados, olives, nuts, and seeds.

Try to include some of these foods in your diet every day. But don't overdo it—they're still high-fat foods, and calories can add up fast. Think of them as replacements rather than add-ons.

HEART-SMART HABITS

Instead of topping a salad with chicken and cheese, opt for avocado and sunflower seeds. If you're worried about protein, throw in some cooked beans.

Avocados, Olives, Nuts, and Seeds

When it comes to good fats, these nutrient-dense plant foods are the best of the bunch. Experiment with each of them to see what you like. Just remember to eat them in small quantities.

Avocados: Avocados are a rich source of both monounsaturated fat (which makes up about 50 percent of the fruit's fat content) and polyunsaturated fat. Plus, they are high in fiber, vitamin C, vitamin K, vitamin E, vitamin B_6, folate, magnesium, and potassium. Similar to leafy greens, avocados also have leutein and zeaxanthin, two plant compounds proven to protect eye health. Half an avocado (about 3½ ounces) has about 160 calories, 15 grams of heart healthy fats, and only 2 grams of saturated fat.

Mashed or puréed avocados are great as spreads in place of fatty mayonnaise. You can also use them on top of chicken, fish, tofu, or vegetables instead of cream sauces. Sliced avocado is a good alternative to cheese on sandwiches and a perfect topping for salads.

Olives: Like avocados, olives are loaded with monounsaturated fat and are most well known for their oil. They are a staple in Mediterranean cuisine, where they are often eaten as snacks. In addition to providing the benefits of olive oil, olives give you fiber, iron, vitamin E, and copper. Since olives are "cured," or processed with salt, beware of sodium levels, which can run high.

Although we see only a dozen or so different kinds of olives in this country, there are hundreds of olive varieties worldwide, in all shades of black, purple, and green. Some ways to incorporate olives into your life include roasting them with vegetables, chopping and sprinkling them on salads in place of salt, and marinating them in a small amount of olive oil with orange or lemon zest and herbs.

Nuts: Nuts have high levels of polyunsaturated fats combined with a good dose of monos. With the exception of Brazil nuts, they also have fewer than 3 grams saturated fat per 1 ounce serving. But it's the extras—protein, fiber, magnesium, copper, vitamin E, and other plant compounds—that make a difference.

Much scientific data shows that nuts such as almonds, walnuts, hazelnuts, peanuts, pecans, pistachios, and some pine nuts reduce the risk of heart disease by lowering unhealthy cholesterol. The latest is a 2010 study that pooled the results of 25 nut-consumption clinical trials. People who added 2.4 ounces of nuts to their daily diet decreased their total cholesterol on average by 5 percent, reduced their LDL cholesterol by 7 percent, and improved the ratio of LDL to "good" HDL cholesterol by 8 percent. Those with high triglycerides saw a drop of more than 10 percent. And researchers think it's more than just the good fats at work. Depending on the kind, nuts can decrease oxidation of LDL cholesterol, reduce inflammation, and improve the dilation of blood vessels.

HEALTHFUL LIVING

Roasting method doesn't matter. Whether they're oil roasted or dry roasted, nuts have the same amount of fat and calories.

The data for nuts and heart disease is so strong that, in 2003, the U.S. Food and Drug Administration allowed marketers to make the health claim that eating 1.5 ounces of nuts a day (that's about one and a half servings) could reduce the risk of heart disease if part of a diet low in saturated fat and cholesterol, and not high in calories.

Even more than cholesterol and heart disease, research shows that eating nuts can positively impact high blood pressure, metabolic syndrome, diabetes, and abdominal obesity. And despite having a reputation of being high in fat and calories, nuts don't make you gain weight. In fact, weight-loss plans that include nuts in the daily diet produce greater compliance and better results than plans that don't. Part of the reason for this is that nuts make you feel full and satisfied. Another theory says that the body may not totally digest nuts, so not all the calories are absorbed. Either way, nuts work.

Although they are more similar than they are different, each nut has its own unique health benefits. Here is a quick rundown:

- **Almonds:** Highest amount of vitamin E, calcium, and fiber; 1 ounce = 23 almonds
- **Walnuts:** Most omega-3 fats; 1 ounce = 14 walnut halves
- **Pecans:** Richest in total antioxidants and beneficial plant sterols (fats); 1 ounce = 19 pecan halves
- **Peanuts:** Excellent source of niacin and plant protein; 1 ounce = about 28 peanuts
- **Pistachios:** Tops among tree nuts in B_6, copper, potassium, and manganese; high levels of antioxidants, like beta-carotene and lutein; 1 ounce = 49 pistachios
- **Cashews:** Highest in zinc, copper, and iron; 1 ounce = 18 cashews
- **Hazelnuts:** Good source of vitamin E, copper, and manganese; 1 ounce = 21 hazelnuts
- **Brazil nuts:** Highest in selenium and magnesium; 1 ounce = 6 Brazil nuts
- **Pine nuts:** In one serving, has more than 120 percent of the daily value for the trace mineral manganese; 1 ounce = 167 pine nuts

When it comes to eating nuts, the most popular way is right out of hand as a snack. But it's easy to overdo nuts if you're grabbing handfuls instead of portioning them out in a baggie so you know exactly how much you have.

In the kitchen use nuts as a condiment. Toss with vegetables and in stir-frys, sprinkle on top of salads, use ground in sauces (nut butters are good for this), and add to fresh fruit or nonfat yogurt for dessert.

Seeds: Like nuts, seeds are chock-full of heart-healthy unsaturated fats and hard-to-get nutrients like magnesium, manganese, calcium, vitamin E, and iron. They are also high in fiber, lignans (plant compounds with antioxidant qualities), omega-3 fatty acids, and phytosterols, a plant compound similar to cholesterol. All these work to lower cholesterol and reduce your risk of heart disease.

Of the most common seeds, flaxseeds have been shown to provide the most benefit to your heart. In addition to cholesterol, flaxseeds lower blood pressure and reduce inflammation.

Because they go rancid quickly, flaxseeds are best bought in whole form and then ground. If eaten whole, they're more likely to pass through your intestine undigested. Beware, however, that flaxseeds do have a distinct flavor that may take some getting used to. Store in the freezer for best results.

In meals, you can use seeds and nuts interchangeably.

Find Time for Fish

Plenty of reasons exist for eating seafood—it's high in quality protein; low in saturated fat; and rich with beneficial nutrients like vitamin A and some B vitamins. Some fatty varieties are also a good source of vitamin D, selenium, and omega-3 fatty acids, a type of fat that boosts heart health.

Omega-3 fatty acids are a type of polyunsaturated fat that is essential, meaning that your body can't produce it and you have to get it from your diet. Three types of omega-3 fatty acids exist: *docosahexaenoic acid (DHA)*, *eicosapentaenoic acid (EPA)*, and *alpha-linolenic acid (ALA)*. DHA and EPA are found in all seafood but are highest in cold-water, fatty fish, like salmon, sardines, herring, mackerel, albacore tuna, and lake trout. ALA is found only in plant sources, like seeds, nuts, leafy greens, tofu, and oils like soybean and canola oil.

DEFINITION

Docosahexaenoic acid (DHA) and **eicosapentaenoic acid (EPA)** are two types of omega-3 fatty acids (polyunsaturated fats) that are found in fatty fish and have been shown to improve heart health. **Alpha-linolenic acid (ALA)** is a type of omega-3 fatty acid (polyunsaturated fat) found only in plant foods, like vegetable oils, seeds, and nuts. In the body, it is partially converted to EPA and DHA, so you have to eat a lot to get the same amount in fish.

Of those, the two most important are DHA and EPA. Why are they so special? When it comes to heart health, few foods compare to the benefits you get from DHA and EPA. Years of research show that these two fatty acids lower total cholesterol, reduce triglyceride levels, ease inflammation, improve blood vessel function, reduce blood clotting, and lower the risk of irregular heartbeats. Then in 2006, Harvard scientists analyzing 20 years' worth of studies concluded that consuming just two to three servings of fish a week could cut the risk of death from heart disease by 36 percent and overall death by 17 percent; they also claimed that the health benefits of eating seafood far outweigh any risk of environmental pollutants such as mercury poisoning.

Based on this evidence and more, the 2010 Dietary Guidelines now recommend that you eat at least two servings of fish (preferably fatty fish) a week. The TLC diet follows the same advice.

More recently, a 2011 British study reviewing several studies found similar results (a 35 percent reduction in sudden cardiac death and 17 percent fewer fatal coronary events) specifically related to daily intakes of 250 milligrams of DHA and EPA. That's exactly what you get if you eat 8 to 12 ounces of seafood a week.

In addition to boosting heart health, omega-3 fats are good for your brain and help fight depression, dementia, and Alzheimer's disease.

Healthy Oils

All fats are composed of three fatty acids: monounsaturated fats, polyunsaturated fats, and saturated fats. How we classify them depends on which fat is most prevalent. Monounsaturated and polyunsaturated fats are called "good" fats because they reduce "bad" LDL cholesterol levels and lower total cholesterol.

Since vegetable oils are liquid at room temperature, they are classified as either monounsaturated or polyunsaturated. Monounsaturated oils include olive oil, canola oil, peanut oil, safflower oil, sesame seed oil, and nut oils.

Of those, olive oil is the most well known and the one with the most famous heart-healthy benefits. Extra-virgin olive oil, the least processed, is chock-full of antioxidants, anti-inflammatory agents, and compounds that can lower LDL and raise HDL.

One of the most potent compounds is oleocanthal, an anti-inflammatory agent that gives you the sting in the back of your throat after you swallow olive oil. It is found in high-quality extra-virgin olive oil and protects against heart disease and dementia. Eating 3 to 4 tablespoons of extra-virgin olive oil containing oleocanthal has been shown to have the same protective power as taking a daily baby aspirin. Although this large amount of olive oil is not recommended here, it is common in certain regions of the Mediterranean.

Polyunsaturated oils are corn oil, sunflower oil, soybean oil, cottonseed oil, and combinations of these; as a group, they're often called vegetable oils or salad oils. Like monounsaturated oils, polys lower LDL cholesterol and reduce your risk of heart disease, but here polyunsaturated fats seem to have an edge over monos mostly because their impact is greater. A 2010 analysis study found that, for every 5 percent increase in calories from polyunsaturated fats (while still reducing saturated fat), heart disease risk dropped by 10 percent.

So which oil should you choose? It's up to you. Since both monos and polys are beneficial for heart health, you might want to consider having both in your pantry.

HEART-SMART HABITS

When it comes to choosing the right oil, let your taste buds be your guide. Many people prefer neutral oils for sautéing and more flavorful oils for salad dressings. Your best bet is to keep several oils in your pantry and use them according to what you are making.

If you buy flavorful oils, think about them more like seasoning ingredients than fats. Think about drizzling them on salads, vegetables, and whole grains to increase flavor or enhance other herbs and spices.

How Much Is Enough?

Many people struggle with the amount of fat they have in their diet. While these fats do offer health benefits when eaten in moderation, more is not better. Also remember that if you up your intake of fat, you need to compensate for it in food later in the day so you don't overeat. Here are some guidelines for what counts as a serving on the TLC diet.

Avocados: One serving of an avocado is about 1 ounce (one fifth of an avocado) and weighs in at 50 calories, with 4.5 grams total fat and .5 grams saturated fat.

Olives: Olive serving sizes vary greatly, depending on the size of the olive, so be sure to read labels. Generally, though, five olives is considered one serving. For instance, five kalamata olives is 45 calories, with 4.5 grams of fat, 0 saturated fat, and 260 milligrams of sodium. Use at your discretion.

Nuts: For most nuts, one serving amounts to about 1/4 cup and supplies between 150 and 200 calories. Recommendations are one to two servings a day.

Fish: If you don't have coronary heart disease, you should be eating a variety of fish two to three times a week. If you do have heart disease, you can still fit fish into the TLC diet two or more times a week, as long as you eat a smaller portion (3 ounces or less). Beware of seafood like shrimp that's high in cholesterol.

Seeds: One serving of seeds is about 1 tablespoon. It's okay to include seeds in your diet every day, especially flaxseeds; aim for sprinkling some seeds on your food at least three to four times a week.

Oils: One tablespoon of oil has about 120 calories, so take those calories into consideration when fitting oil into your diet plan. Because you are eating less red meat, poultry, cheese, and dairy products, you have more leeway when it comes to oils. Depending on your diet plan and calorie level, oil intake can run about 2 tablespoons total per day. If you eat more high-fat protein, seeds, or nuts, you may need to adjust this number.

Fats to Stay Away From

Saturated fats are found in fatty animal meats, like beef, pork, lamb, and poultry with the skin. Fish has some saturated fat, too, but it has more good fat than bad. Other saturated fat culprits are cheese, cream, and butter. A few plant-based foods are also high in saturated fat: coconut oil, palm and palm kernel oil, and cocoa butter.

When it comes to trans fats, you can find them in shortening and some margarines.

Both saturated and trans fats are easy to spot in their pure form, but they're harder to identify when mixed with foods. Some of the worst offenders are buttery croissants and muffins, cheese Danish, cakes, cupcakes, frostings, pastries, and fried foods.

Try to keep both your saturated fat and trans fat intakes as low as possible. Here are tips to help you identify the "bad" guys.

Reduce Meat and Dairy

Most of the saturated fat we get in our diet comes from two sources: cheese and full-fat dairy and processed meats like sausage, bacon, and hot dogs. Fatty chicken dishes and fatty meats like ribs also rank up there. The best way to reduce your consumption of saturated fat is to switch to low-fat or nonfat dairy and to treat cheese, meat, and chicken as side dishes rather than the main entrée.

Always choose lean meats and poultry without the skin. I talk more about protein in Chapter 9.

Most people are pretty good at identifying high-fat meats to avoid, like cheeseburgers. Usually the dairy products and fried foods do us in instead. Unfortunately, these foods are our worst culprits when it comes to saturated fat.

Other times, the size of the meal makes it off limits more than the actual ingredients. This routinely occurs in restaurants. In that case, the best thing to do is simply eat half and pack up the rest before you give in to temptation.

Here are a few surprising sources of high saturated fat that you want to limit or even eliminate on the TLC diet:

- Cream soups
- Pizza topped with fatty meats like sausage and pepperoni
- Oversize omelets and salads loaded with cheese
- Fried chicken wings and chicken pieces
- Cheesy dips, even if they are camouflaged with spinach or artichokes
- Most ice cream shakes and specialty ice cream with add-ins
- Alfredo sauces
- Butter sauces
- Deep-fried appetizers (either frozen or from a restaurant)
- Greek and Caesar salads loaded with fatty cheese and heavy dressings

Go Trans Fat Free

Since 2006, when the Food and Drug Administration required listing trans fats on the nutrition label, trans fats have been in the nutrition spotlight. Developed in the late 1800s as an alternative to butter, trans fats in the form of margarine weren't very popular. Not until World War I and World War II did margarine really take off, when butter was rationed and margarine was used to feed the troops. In no time, hydrogenated fats containing trans fats were used in a wide variety of processed foods to increase shelf life and improve taste and texture.

By raising LDL and reducing HDL, trans fats are much more harmful to your heart than saturated fats. Some scientists believe they're one of the major causes behind the rise in heart disease in this country. Thanks to the efforts of public health agencies and government officials, in recent years, trans fats have been taken out of much of our food supply, making it easier to go trans fat free. However, trans fat still shows up in frostings, microwave popcorn, frozen pizzas, biscuits, margarine, cookies, restaurant foods (think fried chicken, fried fish, and fried potatoes), pies, pastries, and cakes.

Your best bet is to remove most, if not all, processed foods from your diet and restrict eating them to special occasions. Your heart will thank you.

Can I Eat ...

Foods high in saturated fats are not common in the plant kingdom, but there are a few exceptions: coconut oil, palm kernel oil, and cocoa butter. With more than 90 percent saturated fat, coconut oil is the highest saturated fat oil we know of. Next comes palm kernel oil, with well over 80 percent saturated fat; later on the list, with a little more than 60 percent saturated fat, is cocoa.

GOTCHA!

Don't confuse palm kernel oil with palm fruit oil (also known as palm oil). They are completely different. Palm oil is 50 percent saturated, while palm kernel oil is over 80 percent saturated.

Most coconut and palm kernel oils are used to give crispness and crunch to supermarket cakes, cookies, and packaged products, and you should be avoiding these products anyway.

Avoiding saturated fat is important; however, some research shows that not all saturated fats raise cholesterol the same way. That's because not all saturated fats are alike. They consist of different fatty acids, depending on their source—plant or animal, dairy or meat, and so on. This means some are less harmful than others.

In addition, some foods contain other beneficial compounds, like antioxidants, that improve health. Together these two factors mean that some foods high in saturated fat may not be as harmful as once thought—in some cases, they could even have some benefits. This is what happened with chocolate, which the TLC diet allows in small amounts; you can find recipes containing chocolate in Part 4 of this book. Preliminary research suggests that other saturated fats, like butter and coconut oil, may also have some redeeming qualities. Right now, though, not enough data supports including those foods on the TLC diet. Here's what we know.

Chocolate

Chocolate is naturally made up of cocoa butter and nonfat cocoa solids. Since more than 60 percent of cocoa butter is saturated fat, it falls squarely in the realm of a food high in saturated fat. However, more than 50 percent of this saturated fat consists of stearic acid. In studies, stearic acid has been shown to have no effect on blood cholesterol levels. Cocoa butter content also varies among the different chocolate products.

The other part of chocolate, the nonfat cocoa solids, are chock-full of healthy antioxidants called flavonoids. In studies, chocolate's powerful flavonoids fight inflammation, maintain a healthy blood pressure, protect the arteries from damaging cholesterol, and improve insulin sensitivity. When it comes to heart disease, chocolate lowers LDL and total cholesterol without affecting HDL, despite having high fat and calorie levels. One recent 2011 Spanish study published in the *British Journal of Medicine* found that people who had the highest intakes of chocolate reduced their risk of cardiovascular disease by one third.

HEART-SMART HABITS

To get the most bang for your buck, choose dark chocolate with 70 percent or more cocoa. Also, have only a small amount, about 1 ounce a day.

Most of these studies focused on dark chocolate, but other chocolate products are also high in flavonoids. The highest levels are found in natural cocoa powder (not Dutch processed), followed by unsweetened baking chocolate. Dark chocolate comes after that.

Butter

High in saturated fat, butter is considered a splurge on the TLC diet, to be enjoyed only a few times a year. While it is often the first to go on cholesterol-lowering diets, it does have some positive attributes. For instance, it is high in vitamin A; contains vitamins E, K, and D; and also has iodine, calcium, and potassium. If you do decide to try some butter, go for organic, grass-fed brands. Organic butter comes from grass-fed cows that have not been given hormones or antibiotics.

Unlike its conventional counterpart, organic butter is rich in omega-3 fatty acids and also contains conjugated linoleic acid (CLA). CLA is thought to possess anticarcinogenic properties and other health benefits.

GOTCHA!

Stay clear of ghee. Ghee is butter that has been heated so that all the water evaporates and the milk solids are caramelized and removed. Sometimes known as clarified butter, ghee is popular in Indian and Pakistani cuisines.

Coconut Oil

With 95 percent saturated fat, coconut oil beats out butter, beef fat, chicken fat, and shortening for the top spot. In fact, it has more saturated fat than any other food we know of. But surprisingly, pure, virgin organic coconut doesn't raise cholesterol as much as you would think, mostly because of its unique composition. Trans fats are still worse.

Virgin coconut oil consists of an unusual blend of short- and medium-chain fatty acids (most fats are long-chain fatty acids). In the body, it raises LDL, or bad cholesterol, but it also boosts HDL, or good cholesterol, more than most other saturated fats. This is part of its positive quality and may be due to other plant compounds we don't know about.

Coconut meat can be occasionally eaten in small amounts.

Unfortunately, most coconut oil that we see in cookies, cereal, salty snacks, and baked goods is hydrogenated or partially hydrogenated, making it doubly bad for you. Cut these products out of your diet completely.

The Least You Need to Know

- An essential component of the TLC diet is to replace most of your saturated fats with unsaturated fats, like monounsaturated and polyunsaturated fats.
- Saturated fats are solid at room temperature and include animal fat, poultry skin, butter, and full-fat cheeses and dairy. Coconut oil, palm kernel oil, and cocoa butter are also high in saturated fat.
- Avocados, olives, nuts, and seeds are considered "good" fats and have beneficial nutrients. You can include small amounts in your diet every day.
- It's easy to get rid of trans fats in the diet by eliminating processed foods, store-bought baked goods, and fatty restaurant foods.
- Because of its high flavonoid content, dark chocolate is allowed on the TLC diet and is a good treat to have on a regular basis.

Be Careful with Carbs

Chapter

5

In This Chapter

- What's the matter with sugar?
- Passing up pasta and other refined grains
- Shedding your sugary drinks
- Making room for fiber

We are a nation surrounded by high-carbohydrate foods—cakes, cookies, muffins, shakes, soft drinks, pasta, and bread. Everywhere you turn, you can find them. Unfortunately, these carbs are not the kind you should be eating. Bad carbohydrates are devoid of nutrients, filled with empty calories, and highly refined and processed. They tend to be sugary desserts and drinks or starchy foods. Good carbohydrates are chock-full of fiber, vitamins, and minerals, not to mention beneficial phytochemicals. They are found in fresh vegetables, fruits, legumes, and whole grains.

In the body, bad carbohydrates are absorbed quickly and increase blood sugar levels. This results in a cascade of reactions that promote our worst chronic conditions—namely, obesity, diabetes, and heart disease. Good carbs, on the other hand, do just the opposite, entering the bloodstream slowly and protecting us from these mainstream maladies.

In this chapter, you'll understand why keeping your heart in good shape means paying attention to the kinds of carbs you eat. As you'll see, you need to avoid more than just sugar. You also need to watch out for refined carbs like bread and pasta *and* choose the right amount of carbs.

Certainly, eating too much of the wrong kind of carb can be detrimental to your health. In fact, eating too much of *any* carb can lead to problems. But when carbohydrates—specifically, *refined* carbohydrates—replace saturated fat in the diet, the results can be disastrous, particularly for your heart.

Here you learn the ins and outs of carbohydrates; why sugars and starches can be even more hazardous to your health than saturated fats; and what kind of carbs you should be eating to live a long, happy, heart-healthy life.

Simple and Refined Sugars

Carbohydrates are classified into two groups, sugars and starches. *Simple sugars* consist of single units called monosaccharides and include glucose, fructose, and galactose. Glucose is also known as blood sugar and is the type of sugar the body uses for energy. Fructose is known as fruit sugar because it is naturally found in fruit. It's also the sweetest of the sugars. Galactose is a component of milk sugar and is the least sweet.

Then there are the disaccharides, also considered simple sugars, which consist of two monosaccharide units. These are the sugars we are most familiar with in food. They include sucrose (table sugar), honey, high-fructose corn syrup, maple syrup, and more. With the exception of lactose, which is glucose plus galactose, and maltose, which is glucose plus glucose, the majority of disaccharides consist of a combination of glucose and fructose and break down roughly into a 50–50 blend. A couple exceptions are agave and apple juice concentrate, which are much higher in fructose than glucose. (See Chapter 8 for more about the many faces of sugar.)

Refined sugars are simple sugars that have been refined or purified during processing. Most sugars added to foods are refined.

DEFINITION

Simple sugars are readily absorbed by the body. They are naturally found in food or are refined by processing. The main ones are sucrose (table sugar), fructose, and lactose. **Refined sugars** are stripped of all nutrients during processing. White table sugar, cane or beet sugar, high-fructose corn syrup, and dextrose are examples of refined sugars.

In your body, simple sugars are broken down and absorbed into the bloodstream quickly, causing a spike in blood glucose levels and stimulating an aggressive insulin response. Insulin is the hormone that clears glucose from the blood and allows the cells to use it for energy. What the cells don't use is converted to fat, so too much sugar can contribute to weight gain. Too much sugar also causes you to have continuously high blood sugar levels, which increase your chances of developing insulin resistance and diabetes, metabolic syndrome, high blood pressure, and, yes, heart disease. In fact, too much sugar is exactly the problem.

The Problem with Sugar

Simple sugars are naturally found in fruit and milk. These natural sugars are perfectly fine bound with fiber and phytochemicals (in the case of fruit) or protein and fat (in the case of milk and milk products). The real problem is our intake of *added* sugars. These are sugars, usually refined, that are added to foods. Added sugars account for the majority of sugar in our diet. Today Americans consume about 22 to 28 teaspoons of added sugar a day. And although that number has decreased a bit in the past few years, it's still way over recommendations. In fact, sugars and sweeteners total about 17 percent of our overall caloric intake daily. This amounts to roughly 475 calories a day from added sugars.

This is three times the amount health professional organizations like the American Heart Association say we should be getting. They recommend no more than 100 calories, or about 6 teaspoons, of added sugar a day for women and 150 calories, or about 9 teaspoons, a day for men.

So why do Americans eat so much sugar—twice the amount of sugar than the worldwide average? Part of this has to do with our big sweet tooth, which is a direct result of the growing prevalence of sugar and sweeteners in our food supply. Over the last few decades, there has been a huge shift in food preference toward sweetness. Not only has the number of foods containing sugar increased, but the level of sweetness has also gone up. Consider the difference in a cinnamon roll 20 years ago versus today's gargantuan cinnamon buns dripping with frosting. And the more sugar you eat, the more sweetness you crave.

Sugar and sweeteners are also not just in sweet foods. Many manufacturers use sugar as a preservative or stabilizer in addition to a flavor boost. Hidden sugars are mainly found in processed foods and fast food and can also add up. Here are a few sources you may not know about: cereal, salad dressing, canned soup, fruit yogurt, peanut butter, whole-wheat bread, and ketchup (for every 1 tablespoon of ketchup, there is 1 teaspoon of sugar).

GOTCHA!

What is one of the top culprits when it comes to hidden sugars? Tomato sauce. Manufacturers regularly add sugar to balance the acidity of the tomatoes. Though brands vary, most companies add about 1 teaspoon of sugar (4 grams) per $\frac{1}{2}$ cup serving. Remember, tomatoes contain another 5 grams of natural sugar. To avoid this extra sugar, choose brands with no sugar or less sugar added.

What's the best way to take control of your sugar cravings? Cut the sugar completely. This works best if you eat a lot of sugary, sweet foods, but it may be a bit harder if most of your sugars come from fast food and processed foods. Either way, breaking a sugar habit can take weeks or even months, but eventually, you won't even miss the sugar. Furthermore, your sweetness threshold will decrease, meaning that foods that didn't taste sweet before will be kicked up a notch.

Here are some tips to reduce your sugar:

- Choose unsweetened or low-sugar drinks, like tea or sparkling water.
- Eat your fruit *au naturel*, without adding any sugar.
- Use unsweetened applesauce.
- Use fruits canned in natural fruit juice (no sugar added).
- In baking, try cutting the sugar in cookies, brownies, and cakes by one third or one half.
- In desserts, experiment with sweet spices like cinnamon or nutmeg, and extracts like vanilla or almond to bump up flavor without adding sugar.
- Read labels, and avoid frozen vegetables or entrées with added sugar.
- Make your own tomato sauce and soups, without sugar.

Empty Calories

Empty-calorie foods are high in calories but contribute little protein, vitamins, or minerals. A diet high in sugary foods and drinks is high in empty calories. Eating too many empty calories leads to weight gain, particularly around the waist, and an unhealthy diet. On the TLC diet, you'll be replacing empty-calorie foods with low-calorie, high-nutrient foods.

Belly fat increases your risk of metabolic syndrome, diabetes, and heart disease more than fat located in other places, like your butt and your legs. The reason for this is partly location (this fat is closer to your internal organs, like the heart) and partly because of the type of fat. It promotes inflammation, oxidation, and other harmful reactions.

Just as important as how much you eat is what empty calories replace. Filling up on sugary doughnuts and cookies means you have less room for more nutritious foods, like vegetables and beans. This also holds true for beverages like soft drinks and sports drinks. Thus, a diet may be low in saturated fat and cholesterol but still be considered a poor diet because it's high in empty calories, like soft drinks.

Sugar and Heart Disease

Most people don't think of sugar as something to watch for when it comes to heart health, but it is. More scientific evidence is showing that decreasing your sugar intake is an important factor for keeping heart disease at bay.

This evidence, coupled with the fact that intake for soft drinks and sugar-sweetened beverages, our primary source of sugar in the American diet, has more than doubled over the last 30 years, prompted the American Heart Association to issue the sugar guidelines I mentioned earlier: no more than 100 calories, or 6 teaspoons of added sugar, a day for women, and 150 calories, or 9 teaspoons, a day for men.

HEALTHFUL LIVING

Americans consume more soda than any other country in the world, and men drink more soda than women. Per capita, this averages out to almost a gallon a week, or about 45 gallons per year, per person.

What's so bad about sugar? Studies show that, in addition to prompting weight gain, high-sugar diets increase blood pressure, elevate triglycerides, and raise the risk of diabetes, stroke, and metabolic syndrome. All are risk factors for heart disease.

Recent studies focusing on soft drinks found an even stronger link. Based on questionnaires tracking the health of more than 90,000 women from the Nurse's Health Study over two decades, researchers found that women who drank two servings (about 16 ounces) of a sugary beverage per day had a 40 percent higher risk of heart attack or death by heart disease than those who rarely drank sugary drinks.

A newer study presented at the American Heart Association meeting in 2011 showed that middle-aged and older women who drank just two or more sweetened beverages a day were nearly four times as likely to develop high triglycerides and significantly more likely to increase their waist size than those who drank one or less daily. They also developed impaired glucose levels. Surprisingly, the women's waists got bigger even if they didn't gain weight.

What does this mean? Drinking sugary beverages on a regular basis increases a woman's risk for heart disease, metabolic syndrome, and type 2 diabetes, independent of weight gain.

Men face a similar risk when it comes to sugars. In a 2012 study, Harvard researchers followed the diet of more than 40,000 men for 20 years. The men who drank just one 12-ounce sugary beverage a day were 20 percent more likely to get heart disease than their non-soda-drinking counterparts. They also had higher triglyceride levels and lower "good" HDL levels. Less frequent consumption—twice a week or twice a month—didn't increase risk.

But it's not just soda to blame. People who regularly drink sodas are also more likely to follow a typical Western diet—filled with pizza, fast food, and meat—and to be more sedentary. None of those foods are good for your heart.

Sugar and Diabetes

While sugary foods do not cause type 2 diabetes, they certainly contribute to the development of this condition. Over the years, our intake of concentrated sweets and sugars, particularly in the form of beverages, has skyrocketed. The incidence of diabetes has doubled in the last 30 years and is still climbing. Much research has linked these two trends, mainly related to weight gain. And while obesity is still a risk factor for developing diabetes, regularly drinking and eating sugary foods can also raise your chances of getting this condition—even without weight gain.

A review of nearly a dozen studies concluded that people who drink one or two sugary drinks daily are 26 percent more likely to develop diabetes than those sipping less than one a month. Risk of metabolic syndrome also goes up by 20 percent.

Women are particularly susceptible, probably because they require fewer calories than men. Studies show that women who drink one to two servings of sugar-sweetened drinks, including fruit juice, daily are twice as likely to develop type 2 diabetes than those who rarely have these beverages.

Consider that just one 12-ounce can of soda contains about 10 to 12 teaspoons of sugar, and most people gulp that down in just a few minutes. In most healthy people, the body can handle this blast of sugar just fine, but for people who can't manage their glucose as well, this can spell trouble. Furthermore, drinking this much sugar consistently over years is likely to wear down your body's ability to process it, increasing your chances of insulin resistance and, eventually, full-blown diabetes.

HEALTHFUL LIVING

Some ethnic groups have a bigger sweet tooth than others. Latinos and African Americans are more likely to consume sugar-sweetened beverages on a daily basis than Caucasians.

Rein in the Refined Carbohydrates

Refined carbohydrates are carbohydrates that have been processed or modified to enhance shelf life and make them easier to eat or digest. This usually means that they have some part, usually the bran and germ, removed. Refined carbohydrates supply a concentrated source of calories with only a few nutrients. These are usually the white foods: white flour, white rice, white bread, and white sugar. They are generally most prevalent in processed foods and fast food.

On the TLC diet, refined carbohydrates are kept to a minimum. Why? First, because they lack fiber and other nutrients, like trace minerals. Fiber and minerals like magnesium and calcium are particularly good for your heart and your health in general. Second, refined carbs are often found in fast foods and processed foods, like frozen dinners, which tend to be high in fat, calories, and salt. Finally, refined carbs are easy to overeat. Many restaurants use these cheap carbs to fill up plates—think of baskets of bread, plates of pasta, and bowls of rice—and at home, it's just as easy to do the same.

DEFINITION

Refined carbohydrates are carbohydrates that have a part of the food, usually the bran and germ, removed during processing.

Worse Than You Think

Getting the majority of your carbohydrates from refined carbohydrates is not a good idea: you end up missing out on many important vitamins and minerals. But when it comes to heart disease, these carbs can do double damage, especially when they replace saturated fat in the diet.

Until recently, most researchers didn't pay much attention to carbohydrates in the diet. In the last few years, however, more evidence is showing that what you replace saturated fat with is just as important—and may be even more important than lowering saturated fat in general. Several observational and clinical trials concluded that when saturated fat is replaced with polyunsaturated fat, blood cholesterol levels drop and incidence of cardiovascular disease decreases.

When saturated fat is replaced with monounsaturated fat, the effect is more neutral, although there is some benefit. But when saturated fats are replaced by refined carbohydrates, triglyceride levels rise, HDL levels decrease, and LDL cholesterol levels increase. Overall, risk of cardiovascular disease significantly goes up.

Choosing Smart Carbs

Whereas refined carbohydrates may be bad for our heart, other complex carbohydrates are not. These are the carbs found in fruits, vegetables, legumes, and whole grains. Combined with fiber, vitamins and minerals, and beneficial phytochemicals, carbs from these foods are more helpful than harmful. How do you know the difference between good carbs and bad carbs? Here's a list to help you.

Choose more:

Vegetables, especially leafy greens, broccoli, peas, carrots, cabbage, cauliflower, peppers, tomatoes, and onions

Fruits like blueberries, strawberries, blackberries, raspberries, and citrus

Whole-grain bread, pasta, rice, and cereal

Stay away from or limit:

Starchy veggies, like corn and potatoes

Sweetened, syrupy fruits

Refined fruit desserts

Fast food and processed food

Processed white bread, white rice, sugary cereals, and white pasta

Beware of Liquid Calories

Most of us drink more than 22 percent of our total calories. On a 2,000-calorie diet, that comes to about 400 calories—twice the amount nutritionists recommend. It's also more than 50 percent of the added sugars we consume daily.

The lion's share of these calories comes from high-fructose corn syrup or, to a lesser extent, sugar. Both are similar in composition: in high-fructose corn syrup, 55 percent fructose, 45 percent glucose; in sugar, 50 percent fructose, 50 percent glucose. Both are equally bad, although scientists don't agree on exactly how these sugars affect the body. We do know that too much sugar of any kind is not good for you.

In the body, fructose is converted to energy almost exclusively in the liver. When the liver gets overloaded with fructose, it begins to convert this sugar to fat. Some of this fat spills out into our blood as triglycerides. Elevated triglycerides after a meal are the hallmark of a high-fructose (high-sugar) diet.

Elevated triglycerides aren't the only thing fructose fosters, either. It may induce fat accumulation around the liver, which leads to harmful changes in the way the liver manages sugar and fat. It may also cause increased blood pressure and accumulation of visceral fat, both of which are risk factors for metabolic syndrome.

Much of the attention on sugar—particularly fructose—centers on high-fructose corn syrup. While plenty of other sugars are similar to high-fructose corn syrup, high-fructose corn syrup is the one that has been singled out. This is partly because, as a cheap, easy-to-make sweetener, high-fructose corn syrup is rampant in our food supply and appears in most manufacturer products. It's also partly because high-fructose corn syrup is so highly processed and is not naturally found in food (thus, we don't know what its effects are long term). Nevertheless, it is important to avoid all sugar-sweetened beverages, whether they contain high-fructose corn syrup or not. In fact, drinks loaded with beet sugar and cane sugar are no better.

GOTCHA!

Fruit juices are only minimally better for you than soda, largely because not all fruit juices contain the same type or amount of sugar. They also lack fiber and the wonderful phytochemicals whole fruits have.

Mindless Drinking

The biggest problem when it comes to soft drinks and sugar-sweetened drinks is how much we consume. No longer is soda considered a special-occasion treat for Sunday dinner or a special outing. Today it is a part of many people's daily routine. Look around, and you'll see people drinking sodas morning, noon, and night. Many people sip these sweet drinks at their desk throughout the day.

Given the popularity of soft drinks it's not surprising to find that soda now ranks as the top beverage consumed in the United States, beating out milk, water, and juice. But all these soft drinks come with a price: extra calories.

Extra calories would be okay if we made up for them by eating less solid food or exercising more. But we don't. Study after study shows that people do not compensate for liquid calories. The most telling is a study that gave 15 people 450 calories' worth of jelly beans or soda for four weeks. They were then allowed to eat their normal meals. When given the jelly beans, subjects automatically adjusted their intake, eating less solid foods. But when given the soda, they made no such adjustment. After a month, the subjects gained $2\frac{1}{2}$ pounds.

Why don't liquids fill us up? Probably because, for most of man's existence, zero-calorie water was our primary thirst quencher. If man filled up on this drink, he wouldn't survive for long.

Furthermore, the more sweet things we drink, the more sweet things we crave. Soda only enhances our sweet tooth, causing us to look for sweets in other places as well, like cakes, cookies, and desserts.

More Than Just Soda

Soft drinks aren't the only sweet beverages we drink, either. With the advent of specialty coffees and coffee shops, high-calorie drinks like frappuccinos, café mochas, and caramel macchiatos have become common for many people. Most of these drinks are more like glorified flavored shakes and can set you back anywhere from 250 to 550 calories. When it comes to sugar, one of these 16-ounce beverages can run from 32 grams to a whopping 70 grams of sugar (that's nearly 18 teaspoons of sugar).

Bottled sweetened tea is another industry that has benefited from our sweet tooth. Many bottled teas are no different than soft drinks when it comes to sugar. The good news is, both tea and coffee can easily be prepared or bought plain and unsweetened, with no added sugar or fat. My advice is to order tea and coffee straight, without any extras.

Despite their popularity, however, coffee and tea aren't our favorite sugar-sweetened drinks. The top three major sources of added sugars in our diet are sodas, energy drinks, and sports drinks.

HEART-SMART HABITS

If you like your drinks sweet, add sugar yourself so that you control the amount. One packet of sugar is equivalent to 1 teaspoon and contains only 16 calories.

Don't Do Diet (Sodas)

Much controversy surrounds diet sodas and their effect on health. We do know that diet sodas alone do not promote weight loss. In fact, since their emergence into the beverage world in the 1970s obesity has risen, not dropped.

Many theories address this as well, but the main one revolves around the issue that artificial sweeteners are several hundred times sweeter than natural sugars, like sucrose. Although diet sodas do not contain any calories, they do raise our tolerance for sweetness, boosting sweetness levels. Some evidence also indicates that people who drink diet sodas crave more sugary foods (more than people who drink regular sodas). Thus, people who drink diet soft drinks are more likely to be overweight than people who don't drink them.

Weight gain isn't the only thing diet soft drinks have been linked to. Studies also suggest that these drinks increase the risk for metabolic syndrome, diabetes, high blood pressure, and, more recently, heart disease.

The newest and most important study here in this area was conducted by the University of Miami and Columbia University and published early in 2012. Researchers followed more than 2,500 New Yorkers and found that those who drank diet sodas daily were 43 percent more likely to suffer from a vascular event—heart attack, stroke, or vascular death—than those who drank none.

HEART-SMART HABITS

Even if your diet is a good one, it is well worth your while to cut sweet drinks out of your diet. A study from the University of North Carolina at Chapel Hill found that even people who followed a "prudent" (healthful) diet had a higher risk of metabolic syndrome if they drank diet soft drinks than those who didn't drink any diet drinks.

Beverages to Have on Hand

Despite our penchant for sugary drinks, quenching your thirst doesn't have to mean downing spoonfuls of sugar. In fact, there are plenty of really good drinks on the market that are not drowning in sweetness. These include low-fat or nonfat milk, unsweetened almond milk, unsweetened soy milk, 100 percent all-natural juice drinks (on occasion), plain coffee, plain tea, and water, either sparkling or otherwise.

So what are the best drinks to drink on the TLC diet? Here is a roundup.

Water

Of all the nutrients in our diet, water is the most important; it's also the one that's most underappreciated. Water is essential to all our life processes. It is a major component of blood, keeps the blood flowing smoothly, is involved in nearly all reactions in the body, and transports oxygen, vitamins, minerals, and waste.

Most of our water comes from the food we eat. This is particularly true on the TLC diet because of the emphasis on vegetables and fruits, both high-water-content foods. Still, it's good to stay hydrated and sip water throughout the day. Although your water needs vary depending on temperature (you need more when it's hot) and activity levels, most experts advise roughly six to eight glasses of water per day. However, if you feel like this is too much, feel free to dial it down a few notches.

What is one way to know whether you're drinking enough? Check the color of your urine. If it's light yellow, you're getting enough water.

Coffee and Tea, Please

If you're a coffee lover, perk up. Several studies suggest that coffee may have a slight protective effect on the heart. Much of coffee's bad reputation stems from its caffeine content, which was thought to cause a greater risk of heart arrhythmia, but these studies haven't panned out; in fact, some suggest that coffee drinkers may have fewer heart rhythm disturbances than non–coffee drinkers.

Newer studies show that moderate coffee consumption (two to four cups a day) can lower your risk of heart disease by 20 percent. Other studies have shown a lower risk of death from heart disease in coffee drinkers versus non–coffee drinkers. Plus, there may be other benefits: coffee drinking may protect against stroke and type 2 diabetes, gallstones, and liver and colon cancer, as well as lower cholesterol and inflammation levels.

When it comes to heart disease, tea performance is even stronger. Drinking more than six cups of tea day has been associated with a 36 percent lower risk of heart disease. Green tea, in particular, offers short-term improvement in the health of arteries.

But black tea has benefits, too, and also has been shown to lower the risk of heart disease.

Most of these advantages are related to the wealth of antioxidants and unique phytochemicals found in each of these beverages. Brewed beverages, in particular, are much better than bottled—and always choose unsweetened ones.

The bottom line: if you aren't already a coffee drinker, don't think you have to start. In sensitive people, coffee can cause heart palpitations and aggravate conditions like GI reflux, sleep problems, and migraines. If you do drink coffee, keep your intake to around two to four cups a day (don't up it if you're not at that level).

If you're a tea drinker instead, drink a variety of teas. Green, oolong, and black teas all have unique benefits. Always choose brewed and unsweetened or slightly sweetened teas. Tea is not only chock-full of phytochemicals known for their anti-inflammatory, anticarcinogenic, and anti-plaque-forming properties, but it can also curb your appetite, making it a great weight-loss tool if you're dieting.

HEALTHFUL LIVING

The newest trend in teas is fruit-flavored varieties. Made with dried fruits, these teas offer more phytochemicals with no extra calories. You can experiment by adding smashed fresh fruit or citrus to your own fresh-brewed tea.

What About Alcohol?

You may have heard that moderate drinking can potentially protect you from heart disease. This is true. Small amounts of any alcohol could possibly raise HDL, lower blood pressure, inhibit the formation of blood clots, and help prevent artery damage. But the key here is size. *Small* means moderate drinking, which is no more than one drink a day for women and two drinks a day for men. One drink is 12 ounces of beer or a wine cooler, 5 ounces of wine (red is better for your heart than white), or $1\frac{1}{2}$ ounces of 80-proof liquor.

But if you don't drink alcohol already, don't start—and certainly don't drink more than the recommendation. Drinking too much alcohol has many harmful effects. It can damage the heart and arteries, raise blood pressure, and increase triglycerides.

And don't forget that alcohol has calories, so if you're trying to lose weight, you'll want to avoid alcoholic drinks.

High-Fiber Heroes: Complex Carbohydrates

Unlike simple carbohydrates, complex carbs are large molecules that the body absorbs more slowly. They fall into two camps, depending on their digestibility, size, and structure: starches and fibers. High-fiber complex carbohydrates like fresh fruits, vegetables, legumes, and whole grains are preferred, since many starchy carbohydrates like breads and pastas are refined.

Current fiber intakes in the typical American diet are low, about half of what you'll eat on the TLC diet. This is mainly due to our reliance on processed foods, but since you'll be eating a lot more vegetables, fruits, and whole grains, this won't be a problem. As long as you can tolerate it, the more fiber you eat, the better—in the form of fruits, vegetables, whole grains, and a variety of foods. Currently, there is no upper limit or cap set on the amount of fiber we can consume.

Soluble vs. Insoluble and Resistant Starch

Two types of fiber are found in foods, soluble fibers and insoluble fiber. All foods contain both types of fibers; we just classify them according to the one that's most dominant.

Soluble fibers include pectin and gums. Found in plant cells, they absorb water and expand during digestion, which is why you feel full after eating them. They help your body make bulkier, softer stools and are particularly important for heart health. Soluble fibers absorb cholesterol in the form of bile, which breaks down fat. This cholesterol is most likely to be the form of LDL cholesterol. Once it's bound to fiber, the cholesterol is swept through the system and is eventually excreted into the stool. Typically, bile is recycled and ends up back in the digestive system.

If the body is continuously excreting bile acids, the liver needs to make more, pulling LDL cholesterol out of the bloodstream. This is one way high-fiber foods lower LDL and total cholesterol levels in the blood.

Since soluble fiber is so important for lowering cholesterol, the TLC diet recommends that you get at least 5 to 10 grams of soluble fiber a day—and preferably 10 to 25 grams a day to lower LDL cholesterol. I'll talk more about soluble fiber in Chapter 14.

Insoluble fibers come from the cell walls of plants and include cellulose and lignin. Like soluble fiber, they are not digested, but rather pass through the digestive system. These fibers speed up the movement of food through the digestive tract and keep things rolling smoothly. Like soluble fiber, insoluble fiber lowers cholesterol, but the mechanism by which it does this is not exactly clear.

Best Bets for Complex Carbs

On the TLC diet, you'll be eating 20 to 30 grams of fiber per day. It's okay to eat more than that, as long as you have no problems tolerating it and eat a wide variety of foods. In fact, most of the higher-calorie menus in this book have between 35 and 45 grams of fiber, thanks to the emphasis on fruits, vegetables, and whole grains. Generally the more calories you eat, the more fiber you'll get.

For the most part, however, the issue is not getting enough fiber. Consequently, you need to home in on high-fiber foods. You'll find fiber throughout the plant kingdom, but it is most prevalent in beans, which provide about 6 to 8 grams of fiber per serving. Beans are a good source of soluble fiber, as are many fruits like citrus and pears. Still, vegetables are no slouches in this department, and whole grains are also big fiber-filled foods. You can't always tell how much fiber is in a food by looking at it, either. For instance, a crunchy carrot and a piece of celery have only about 2 grams of fiber each, but $\frac{1}{2}$ cup green peas has 9 grams of fiber, and $\frac{1}{2}$ cup cooked spinach has 7 grams.

GOTCHA!

Increase the amount of fiber in your diet slowly, to keep from experiencing any abdominal cramps or bloating. Remember, your body may need an adjustment period of a few weeks.

Whenever possible, eat the whole food, including skin and seeds. Don't peel carrots, cucumbers, or apples. Here are some tips on choosing good high-fiber foods:

- Choose whole grains, like brown rice, oatmeal, quinoa, and pearled or unhulled barley over refined grains.
- Eat more beans and dried peas, especially lentils, split peas, black beans, red beans, chickpeas, and lima beans.
- Load up on cruciferous vegetables, like broccoli, brussels sprouts, cauliflower, and dark leafy greens.
- Bask in berries, including strawberries, raspberries, blueberries, and blackberries.
- Other fruits, like pears, avocados, and apples, are also good sources of fiber.

Keep in mind that fiber is only one of the many beneficial plant compounds in fruits, vegetables, and grains that will keep you and your heart healthy and strong. These foods also contain potent antioxidants and hundreds of compounds that enhance the immune system and keep the body strong and healthy. That's why it's important to focus on the whole food rather than just one part.

The Least You Need to Know

- Too much sugar in the diet, especially in the form of soft drinks and sugar-sweetened beverages, not only can harm your heart, but also increases your chances of getting diabetes, metabolic syndrome, and high blood pressure.
- When it comes to heart health, you want to lower saturated fat and replace it with polyunsaturated fat. If you lower saturated fat and increase refined carbohydrates, you increase your risk of heart disease.
- The major source of added sugars in the diet comes from sugar-sweetened drinks like soft drinks, energy drinks, and sports drinks. Diet soft drinks are no better.
- Drinking moderate amounts of coffee, tea, and alcohol is allowed on the TLC diet and may even offer some health benefits for your heart.
- High-fiber, complex carbohydrates have many benefits. Soluble fiber found in vegetables, whole grains, and fruits are good carbs that remove cholesterol from the bloodstream and reduce the risk of cardiovascular disease.

Chapter 6

Watch the Salt

In This Chapter

- How much salt do we need?
- The problem with salt
- Surprising sources of sodium
- Salty habits to break

We all know too much salt is not good for us. But that doesn't stop us from piling it on. We like salty foods (french fries are a favorite), salty snacks, and even salty desserts. Something about salt is just so appealing. It not only tastes good, but it enhances the flavor of food. This is why some people find it so hard to give up salt.

But lowering salt intake is a good practice for everyone, young and old. Reduce the salt in your diet, and your heart, arteries, kidneys, and bones will thank you. Here we explain why high salt intakes are associated with high blood pressure, kidney stones, and osteoporosis, and we briefly review the science behind it.

Since you're concerned about your heart and your health, you've probably already ditched most salty foods. Chances are, you may have even given up the salt shaker. That's good, but for most people on the TLC diet, that's just not enough. Much of the salt in our food supply is hidden in foods that don't taste salty. In this chapter, I tell you how to recognize those foods and why it's important to make smart choices. I also give you suggestions on how to break the salt habit. But don't be afraid that your food will taste bland. I discuss plenty of ways to season your meals with fresh herbs and spices so that it will taste so bright, clean, and delicious. You won't even miss the salt … eventually.

How Much Is Enough?

When it comes to salt, we're most concerned about sodium. Sodium is a major mineral that the body requires. It's essential in our diet, meaning we have to get it in food. While too much sodium can cause problems in the body, too little is also bad. Many people use the terms *salt* and *sodium* interchangeably. They are not the same thing.

Salt consists of 40 percent sodium and 60 percent chloride. Thus, a low-salt diet is less restrictive than a low-sodium diet. Sodium levels are what nutrition food labels list, in milligram amounts. Sodium levels are also how most health professionals and organizations characterize low-salt diets. One teaspoon of salt contains a little more than 2,300 milligrams of sodium. This is about your limit for a total day, according to the 2010 Dietary Guidelines.

Although sodium is found in other forms than sodium chloride, salt is definitely the most common. That's why when we talk about reducing sodium, we often refer to it as salt.

GOTCHA!

Other forms of sodium in the diet include sodium bicarbonate (baking soda), sodium acid pyrophosphate (baking powder), monosodium glutamate (MSG), sodium alginate, disodium phosphate, sodium nitrate, and nitrite. The last four are used in processed foods like ice cream, pudding, gravy, and cured meats to preserve, thicken, emulsify, or cure foods.

Having Salt Sense

In the body, salt is broken down into its two main components, sodium and chloride. Chloride helps maintain fluid balance in the body and is a necessary component for digestion and absorption. Specifically, chloride is part of a compound in your stomach known as hydrochloric acid. This acid breaks down food.

Sodium has several main functions: it regulates blood volume, maintains acid-base balance in the blood, is required for normal muscle contractions and nerve impulses, and helps the body absorb glucose and amino acids during digestion.

Surprisingly, we don't need much of it to survive. In fact, all we need is 200 milligrams to maintain normal physiological function. Current recommendations, also called adequate intakes, support good health and are much more generous than that.

According to the 2010 Dietary Guidelines, adolescents and adults age 50 years and younger (to age 14 years) would do best to keep their sodium intake at 1,500 milligrams per day, with an upper limit of no more than 2,300 milligrams of sodium daily. Indeed, the goal of getting *less than 2,300 milligrams daily* is the one touted by almost all health professionals. Lower levels are set for young children and older adults.

Nevertheless, despite these high sodium levels, much controversy still surrounds exactly how much salt we should be having or can have on a healthy diet. Salt proponents say salt is not to blame for other health problems and cite studies supporting their position. Still, major health professional organizations and the weight of scientific evidence leans in favor of reducing sodium intake as much as possible.

On the TLC diet, you should aim for less than 2,300 milligrams of sodium daily unless you are older than 51 years of age; are African American (at any age); or have high blood pressure, diabetes, or chronic kidney disease. In these cases, the upper limit of sodium is set at 1,500 milligrams. All the TLC menus in this book are designed to have less than 2,300 milligrams of sodium; however, some fall below the 1,500 mark as well simply because they focus on whole, natural, unprocessed foods.

HEART-SMART HABITS

Because of its relationship to heart disease, the American Heart Association recommends that all people who are concerned about heart health limit their sodium intake to less than 1,500 milligrams of sodium per day.

Current Intakes

So how far off the mark are we? Pretty far. According to the Centers for Disease Control and Prevention (CDC), more than 90 percent of Americans eat more sodium than is recommended for a healthy diet. The amount we're consuming? About 3,300 to 3,400 milligrams of sodium a day. This translates into about $1\frac{1}{2}$ teaspoons of salt a day. That's about 50 percent more than the USDA Dietary Guidelines and the TLC diet recommend.

Keep in mind, too, that this number is an average. I've seen students (on poor diets) easily take in 5,000 or 6,000 milligrams of sodium in a single day, mainly from prepared restaurant food or fast food. Unfortunately, most of my students (and clients as well) are unaware of how much sodium they're taking in, unless it's called to their attention. The good news is, it's easy to get a handle on your salt intake, if you know what to do.

Why Is Salt So Bad?

I get this question often from my students when I teach nutrition, and the answer is simple. Too much sodium in the diet increases your risk of heart attack and stroke, mainly by raising blood pressure, a major risk factor for both of these health outcomes. If that's not enough reason, I also explain that most of the salty foods in our diet are high in fat and calories—not a good combination. Following is an explanation of these reasons and more.

Raises Blood Pressure

Sodium naturally attracts water. When we eat too many salty foods, the sodium in our bloodstream goes up, causing the body to retain water to balance out this concentration. This is why we get thirsty when we eat salty foods. It's also the mechanism behind belly bloat, the swollen belly you get when you eat too much salty food. Eventually, this excess sodium is filtered out of the body through the kidneys.

Having high blood sodium levels makes your blood volume increase. A greater blood volume means your heart is working harder to move the blood through your system. This also increases the pressure in your arteries. Over time, high blood pressure can damage arteries, leading to heart problems or stroke. If you have high blood pressure, you're also at an increased risk for metabolic syndrome.

High blood pressure, or *hypertension*, as it is often called, is known as the silent killer because most people don't know they have it until something happens.

Some people are more *salt sensitive* than others. If you are salt sensitive, your body responds to your dietary salt intake by raising blood pressure. People who are not salt sensitive don't see this effect. It's hard to tell who is salt sensitive and who is not on an individual level, but we do know that certain groups of people in general are more salt sensitive than others. These include older people, African Americans, and people who already have high blood pressure. Some researchers have estimated that about a quarter of the population with normal blood pressure are salt sensitive, and about half of the population with high blood pressure seems to be affected.

DEFINITION

Hypertension is the medical term for high blood pressure (a blood pressure reading of 140 over 90 or greater for either number). **Salt sensitivity** means that the salt you eat in your diet directly raises your blood pressure. Not all people are salt sensitive. People who are salt sensitive are at higher risk for heart attacks, strokes, and metabolic syndrome than people who aren't.

But whether you are salt sensitive or not, lowering your salt intake is still recommended on the TLC diet. A 2010 *New England Journal of Medicine* study done by researchers at the University of California, Stanford, and Columbia University estimated that if Americans reduced their salt intake by a modest 3 grams (about 1,200 milligrams a day), there would be 155,000 fewer heart attacks and strokes annually.

Can Cause Kidney Stones

Anyone who has ever had a kidney stone (or knows someone who has had one) understands how painful and debilitating this condition can be. Kidney stones are small, hard pebblelike crystals that form in the kidney. There are four types: calcium, struvite, uric acid, and cystin. Of those, calcium kidney stones are the most common and the ones related to high-salt diets.

The reason has to do with the fact that high-sodium diets are associated with increased calcium losses. Thus, the more salt you eat, the more salt and calcium are excreted in your urine. If more calcium is excreted, more calcium is circulating in the bloodstream. More calcium in the bloodstream means you have a greater chance of forming calcium kidney stones. It's not a good idea to limit calcium intake, particularly if you're worried about osteoporosis. However, reducing salt intake results in less calcium being lost and a lower chance of developing kidney stones.

Bad for Your Bones

Since high-salt diets lead to higher calcium losses, many experts suspect that a high-salt diet can also put you at risk for osteoporosis. Osteoporosis is a condition characterized by porous and fragile bones. It is caused by a loss of calcium.

As we age, the risk for this disease goes up. Today osteoporosis affects more than 8 million women and 2 million men in the United States. Unfortunately, many people don't know they have it until a break occurs. Low calcium intakes are the main reason for this illness, particularly during the teenage years when we need it the most. Unfortunately, most people don't get enough. Combine this with high-salt diets that increase losses, and the risk is even higher.

High in Fat and Calories

Most of the salty foods in our diet are also high in fat and calories. Unlike Asian cuisines, like Chinese, Japanese, Korean, and Thai—which tend to concentrate their salt in sauces and condiments like fish sauce, soy sauce, and cured or dried fish—American salty foods are more likely to be in the form of fatty meats, cheese, salty snacks, and restaurant foods (think nachos and cheese or tacos). Many of these foods are high in calories, saturated fat, and sodium, making them already off limits on the TLC diet.

Consider some of these popular items:

- Chipotle chicken and cheese burrito with pinto beans, rice, and salsa: 975 calories, 11 grams saturated fat, 2,630 milligrams sodium
- Panera Bread smoked ham and Swiss on rye bread: 590 calories, 8 grams saturated fat, 1,870 milligrams sodium
- Pizza Hut pepperoni pizza (two slices): 500 calories, 9 grams saturated fat, 1,180 milligrams sodium
- Hebrew National quarter-pound hot dog and bun: 470 calories, 13 grams saturated fat, 1,330 milligrams sodium
- Burger King Whopper with cheese: 760 calories, 16 grams saturated fat, 1,410 milligrams sodium

Keep in mind, too, that sodium levels vary greatly even among the same food, depending on how it is made and who makes it. For example, different brands of chicken noodle soup can vary by as much as 840 milligrams of sodium. Your best bet here is to always read the label.

A Taste We Crave

Unlike sweetness, which is a taste we are innately born to like, salt is a taste we learn to like with repeated exposure. Unfortunately, it is also a taste we quickly adapt to. Thus, the more salty foods we eat, the more we become "used" to the taste. Over time, our taste begins to get desensitized or resistant to salt. As a result, we crave more and more. This is the reasoning behind food manufacturers' quest for "extreme" flavor profiles, like Doritos Sizzlin' Cayenne and Cheese Flavored Tortilla Chips, or Cheetos Flamin' Hot Limon Cheese snacks. This is also why some salty foods can taste so salty to one person that they're nearly inedible, while another person finds the taste not salty at all. So accustomed have we gotten to the taste of salt that some people salt their food without even tasting it first.

The good news is, since salt is an acquired taste, we can also "unlearn" it, meaning we can retrain our taste receptors to get used to less salt. Although this can take several weeks (and sometimes even months), studies on taste have shown that our desire for salty foods can be significantly reduced and sometimes even disappear altogether.

Surprising Sources

Many people think all they need to do to reduce their salt intake is to cut out the salt. That's just not true. In fact, according to the CDC, more than 75 percent of the sodium Americans consume comes from processed and prepared foods. *Prepared* means ready-to-eat foods from grocery stores and foods made in restaurants and fast-food outlets. Only 5 to 6 percent of our sodium intake is added at home during cooking, and another 5 to 6 percent is added at the table with the salt shaker. Thus, the lion's share of our sodium intake comes from processed foods.

GOTCHA!

Even if you cut out all added salt and processed food from your diet, you don't have to worry about getting too little sodium. Small amounts of this important mineral are naturally found in meat, milk, and vegetables. Consequently, the TLC diet provides all the sodium you need for good health.

To help people figure out where their salt is coming from, the CDC recently released a report listing the top 10 food sources of sodium in the diet. Together these 10 food groups account for 44 percent of the sodium in a typical U.S. diet. Here is the list the CDC came up with and ways you can reduce your intake.

Bread and rolls. The most startling finding of the CDC analysis is that the majority of our sodium intake comes not from salty snacks or other obvious sources, but from plain old bread. It's not that bread is especially high in sodium—levels range from 80 to 230 milligrams per slice—it's that we eat it several times a day.

What to do: You can buy low-sodium breads; be sure to keep these in the freezer as without salt, bread gets stale faster. Another option is to just watch the amount of bread you're eating. Try not to have more than two or three slices of bread (or one to two rolls) a day.

Cold cuts and cured meats. No surprises here—curing uses tons of salt, and cold cuts are notorious for their high salt content.

What to do: Go for reduced-sodium brands of cold cuts, which can shave off as much as 25 percent sodium from regular brands. Otherwise, try cooking and slicing your meat yourself—this works well with turkey breast. When it comes to cured meats like bacon, look for lower-sodium brands. If you do want the real thing, treat it as a special food to be eaten only once or twice a month.

Pizza. For most people, pizza is another shocker, mostly because it doesn't necessarily taste salty. Consider the high-sodium ingredients: mozzarella cheese, pepperoni (the most popular pizza topping in this country), tomato sauce, and the pizza crust—bread.

What to do: Make it yourself. This gives you the ability to control the toppings, the cheese, and the sauce (homemade is best using "no salt added" tomato sauce) and significantly reduce the sodium. See Chapter 18 for some pizza recipes. If you don't have time to make it yourself, there's not much you can do to pizza to reduce the sodium other than skipping the pepperoni, so your best bet is to just go easy on the portions. Try to stick to one slice; then make a salad or have something else.

Fresh and processed poultry. Most everyone can understand that processed chicken, like chicken nuggets and breaded and fried fillets, are high in sodium, but fresh? Many food manufacturers regularly plump up "fresh" chicken (and pork) by injecting them with a salt solution. This means your typical 45- to 70-milligram sodium chicken can now contain some 300 or 400 milligrams of sodium per serving. Worse yet, you're paying a premium for salt and water.

What to do: Read the fine print and look at the nutrition label. Don't buy anything that says it contains or is "enhanced" with a 15 percent solution chicken broth (or other ingredients).

Soups. Canned soups are loaded with sodium. Even the low-sodium varieties are higher than what you would get if you made soup yourself from scratch.

What to do: Skip the can and make your own soup from scratch. If it's hard to find the time, devote one weekend a month to making soup. Make several big batches and then freeze them. Check out the soup recipes in Chapter 18.

Sandwiches and burgers. Both of these types of foods pack in the sodium. This is partly because of the amount of meat they pile on, which is either treated with a sodium solution or seasoned with salt, and partly because of the sauces and toppings that are added.

What to do: Make your own sandwiches at home so you can control the fat and sodium. If that's not possible, think small. Order junior burgers, kids' meals, or half sandwiches when you can. Also make it plain, skip the cheese and sauce, or order sauce on the side so you can add it yourself.

Cheese. Cheese is inherently salty simply because you need salt to make cheese.

What to do: When it comes to sodium, certain cheese is better than others. For example, Swiss and mozzarella are good choices that are fairly low in sodium, whereas blue cheese and feta are not. Since cheese is high in saturated fat, you'll be having only small amounts of cheese to begin with, so monitoring sodium will be easier.

Pasta mixed dishes. Spaghetti with meat sauce or even marinara can rank pretty high in sodium, due to both the pasta and the sauce. Other pasta and sauces are also high in sodium.

What to do: Make your own sauce using "no salt added" tomato products, if you can. If not, watch the portion size. If you're at a restaurant, don't think you have to eat all of what you're served. Eat half and take the rest home.

Meat mixed dishes. Meat mixed dishes, like pasta dishes, are almost always high in sodium, whether prepared in the grocery store or bought at a restaurant. Think meatballs, meatloaf, beef stew, beef pot pie, tamales, enchiladas, meat lasagna, and empanadas, for example.

What to do: Make your own from scratch, when you can, and go easy on the serving size.

Snacks. Last on the list are salty snacks, like chips, crackers, and pretzels.

What to do: Most of these you'll be removing from your diet anyway, in favor of more healthy vegetables and fruits. Otherwise, choose low-sodium or reduced-sodium versions.

Getting Salt Under Control

Now that you know why too much salt is bad for you and where it is found, it's time to think about how to reduce your intake. Before you start making changes, first figure out exactly where your salt-centered foods are. Do you eat a lot of salty snacks and processed foods? Are you someone who eats out often? Is bread your downfall? Or do you often use salt in cooking? Once you've decided where your salty foods lie, you can come up with a strategy to decrease them. Here's what you need to keep in mind.

Choose Kosher or Sea Salt

As you read earlier, salt added to food at the table is actually the least of your worries. That's because, despite the fact that food tastes saltier, the amount you add to your food is fairly low (only 5 to 6 percent of total salt intake). So if you've cut out all processed convenience and prepared foods and reduced the salt in your cooking, keeping the salt shaker on the table may be okay. But if you're trying to retrain your taste buds and decrease your desire for salt, it's best to go cold turkey and remove salt from the table as well as the kitchen.

If you do want to keep some salt in the house, which one you choose does make a difference. While all salt is the same in composition, it varies in terms of size and shape of crystal. This, in turn, affects how much salt is packed into one teaspoon. Thus, large crystals like kosher salt contain less salt per teaspoon than finely textured sea salt.

HEART-SMART HABITS

If you want to use salt on the table, go for the bigger crystals like kosher salt or sea salt. Kosher salts contain anywhere from one fifth to one half the amount of sodium per teaspoon as in regular fine-grain salts.

If taste is more your concern, think about trying some flavorful sea salts. There are also Himalayan salt, Hawaiian salt, and pink salt. These salts are more expensive, which might also curb usage, and often contain various minerals affecting color and flavor. They also come in a variety of unique shapes and sizes that burst on the tongue, giving a strong salt flavor. Use them as finishing salts on top of soups or salads to add flavor.

Pass on Processed Foods and Dining Out

When it comes to sodium—and saturated fat and calories, for that matter—processed, prepared, or convenience foods and restaurant foods are not something you should be eating on a regular basis. Nearly all of the CDC's top 10 sources of high-sodium foods listed earlier fall into the category of processed or prepared foods. Other high-sodium foods to avoid include these:

- Salad dressings and sauces
- Condiments
- Canned goods, especially chicken and beef broth

- Ready-to-eat cereal
- Pickled foods
- Prepared box mixes of potatoes, rice, and pasta

If you're unsure of what constitutes a processed or prepared food, keep this general rule in mind: any food that comes out of a box, bag, can, or package is processed. These foods include side dishes, like broccoli with cheese sauce, hash browns, or green bean almondine; dinner entrées, like stews, prepared meats, and frozen dinners; appetizers, such as breaded and fried items, mini pizzas, garlic bread, and stuffed potatoes; and, finally, frozen or fresh desserts, such as pies, puddings, cheesecake, and frozen sweets. While you will not always be able to avoid processed foods altogether, if you follow the TLC diet, most likely you'll be hitting the 80/20 rule. This is 80 percent whole, natural, unprocessed food and 20 percent processed. This is a good formula to keep in mind.

If you do buy processed or prepared foods, look for low-sodium or reduced-sodium brands. But be sure to check the label (see Chapter 8). Even if some products claim to be lower in sodium, they may still be high in sodium. This is the case with chicken or beef broths and soy sauce. Using light or low-sodium brands is better than using regular, but keep in mind that they are still high in salt and should be used sparingly.

If you go out to eat often, salt (and fat) can rack up faster than you think. According to the CDC, about 25 percent of our daily sodium intake comes from restaurant foods. Learning to make the right choices when dining out takes time and practice, as well as some knowledge about food and how it is prepared. I talk in more depth about strategies for dining out on the TLC diet in Chapter 12.

Your goal is to cook most of your meals at home from fresh, unprocessed vegetables, grains, and meats, and fish and poultry. View dining out as an occasional treat, to be enjoyed once or twice a month.

Don't Cook with Salt

Reducing the salt you use in cooking is probably one of the easiest ways to lower your salt intake. This is because you have control of how much you use. If you're concerned about how your food will taste, begin slowly, first by reducing salt by only one quarter or one half. Then you can gradually try removing the salt altogether.

The key here is to replace the flavor you lost via the salt by adding more herbs and spices.

HEALTHFUL LIVING

Did you know 75 percent of what we taste is actually a result of smell? Smell allows us to tell the difference between a grapefruit and an orange. For this reason, use the most aromatic herbs and spices you can find in your cooking, and revel in the smell. It makes a difference.

Up Your Herbs and Spices

Using more fresh herbs and dried spices is the best way to perk up bland-tasting food and kick the salt habit. Often people add salt to their food simply because they don't know what other spices or herbs to add. But once you get accustomed to using these seasoning ingredients, the possibilities are endless. Consider the following tricks of the trade to get you started.

Start with your favorite herbs and spices. Some people have their own special herb or spice that they use over and over again. These are what I call "comfort" spices. They are my go-to spices when I don't know what to add in a recipe. For me, they are garlic, basil, onion, and oregano. My spice pantry is never without these ingredients. Someone else might favor other spices or herbs, like parsley, chili powder, coriander, and ginger.

Think about combinations. Some herbs and spices naturally go together—garlic and onion, oregano and lemon, ginger and soy sauce. Write a list of your favorite combinations of spices and herbs, and look at it before you start cooking. If you're not sure where to start, get some food magazines or peruse some cookbooks; go to the library or ask some friends. You may even want to buy a good herb and spice cookbook (there are many, if you just Google them). Another option is to look at food blogs—you can find hundreds of them online. You can also search at foodblogsearch.com, and some great blog search sites, like feastie.com, allow you to bookmark recipes and even create your own set of favorite recipes.

Look to ethnic foods. Many ethnic foods use a variety of herbs and spices. Pick your favorite cuisine, and learn what herbs and spices are most commonly used and how. Some of the countries most noted for their herb and spice dishes are India, Thailand, Korea, Southern France, Sicily, Greece, and Morocco.

Experiment with spicy. Poblanos, jalapeños, New Mexican peppers, habaneros, and ghost peppers are just a few of the many hot peppers made into spices or used fresh. Explore the world of hot and spicy, and you surely will not miss the salt.

Need a little help with your spice pantry? Consider adding these:

- Basil
- Chili powder
- Cinnamon
- Cloves
- Coriander
- Cumin
- Dill weed and dill seed
- Garlic powder
- Ginger
- Marjoram
- Nutmeg
- Onion powder
- Oregano
- Parsley
- Rosemary
- Sage
- Thyme

Pump Up Potassium

High-sodium diets are generally low in potassium. Indeed, the two go hand in hand. Low potassium levels contribute to salt sensitivity and high blood pressure. Studies show that increasing potassium intakes brings blood pressure down and can reduce cardiovascular disease and stroke by improving blood vessel function. It can also improve bone mineral density and lower your chances of getting kidney stones. This is virtually the opposite of what sodium does in the body, and a similar relationship exists in food.

High-sodium, processed foods lack potassium, whereas high-potassium foods—fruits, vegetables, and beans—are generally low in sodium. Thus, improving the ratio of potassium to sodium—in effect, boosting potassium and reducing sodium—is easier than you think. This becomes even more important when you consider that it's associated with improved heart health. Here are some high-potassium foods:

- Bananas
- Cantaloupe and honeydew
- Halibut, rockfish, and cod
- Nonfat milk
- Nonfat yogurt
- Soybeans, lima beans, black beans, and lentils
- Sweet potatoes and white potatoes
- Tomatoes
- Winter squash

Remember, changing your diet is not something you can do overnight. Removing the salt and the fat, adding more herbs and spices, upping your vegetable intake, and eating fewer convenience, prepared foods may take some getting used to. The key to success is making changes in small steps gradually. This will give you and your taste buds time to adjust to this new, healthier way of eating. In the end, your body and your mouth will thank you.

The Least You Need to Know

- Most people eat way too much salt. The TLC diet limits salt intake to less than 2,300 milligrams of sodium a day.
- High-salt diets can increase your chances of having a heart attack or stroke by raising blood pressure and increasing your risk of metabolic syndrome.
- Since the majority of our sodium comes from processed and prepared foods like bread, pizza, and deli meats, the best way to reduce intake is to eliminate convenience foods or choose low-sodium options and limit dining out.
- At home, the best way to "retrain" your taste buds and get used to less salt is to emphasize fresh herbs and spices and avoid cooking with salt.
- Don't worry about getting too little salt. Sodium is naturally found in vegetables, meat, and milk.

Part 2

Everyday Diet Decisions

Now that you know what you should be eating, it's time to actually make some changes and practice what you preach. This part tells you how to clean out your kitchen to make room for healthful TLC food—what to throw out and what to keep. Then it gives you step-by-step guidance on how to navigate the grocery store so you can make good choices and stock a nutritious TLC pantry at home. There's also a chapter just on protein, since this is an area where many people run into trouble.

Chapter 7

Start at Home

In This Chapter

- Creating a heart-smart kitchen
- Having the right tools at hand
- Learning kitchen shortcuts
- Becoming a master menu planner

Good health starts with good nutrition, and good nutrition starts with a good kitchen. Now that you know the basic principles of the TLC diet, it's time to start making changes that will make it easier for you and your family to make healthy choices, especially at home.

The best way to do this is to get rid of fatty, sugary, salty foods that are bad for your health. So get ready to clean out your pantry, fridge, and freezer. Not only does this remove temptation, but it also makes room for the more nutritious foods that you'll now be eating more of. In this chapter, you learn how to reorganize and revamp your kitchen.

Once you get your kitchen in order, you'll find it easier to spend more time in the kitchen cooking healthfully for you and your family. If you don't feel comfortable in the kitchen, take a few classes or cook with a friend. Being able to prepare and plan healthful meals is the cornerstone of the TLC diet.

But don't fret. I give you plenty of tips for making this diet fit into your lifestyle. Whether you're a leisurely cook or someone who likes to get in and out of the kitchen quickly, proper planning is the key to success and the best way to get a quick, healthful, and tasty meal on the dinner table every night.

Clean Out the Kitchen

Most of the foods in the typical American diet are high in fat, saturated fat, cholesterol, and sodium. Consequently, these are also the kinds of foods that fill up our shelves. For this reason, most people switching to the TLC diet need a kitchen overhaul.

Filling your pantry, refrigerator, and freezer with a variety of nutritious, healthful foods is the first step in adopting this lifestyle and can be a huge undertaking for people not used to eating that way. For more energetic people, this means making a clean sweep and jumping right in. Others, who rely more heavily on processed foods, may take a more gradual approach. For them small steps work best, like first upping fruits and vegetables; then reducing fatty meat, fried chicken, and fried fish; then choosing low-fat or nonfat dairy; and so on.

Either way, when it comes to eating a cholesterol-lowering diet high in healthful, low-fat foods, the best strategy for achieving success is "out of sight, out of mind." Remove the offending food, and eventually, you won't even miss it.

Pull Out the Processed Foods

Technically, processed foods are any foods that have been altered or changed from their natural state. In our food supply, this covers a lot of ground. If you think about processed food as any prepared food from a restaurant or fast-food establishment, or any convenience food that comes out of a box, bag, bottle, package, or can, you'll begin to realize just how prevalent these foods are.

From a health standpoint, processed or prepared foods are typically high in saturated fat, cholesterol, and sodium; they also lack fiber, trace minerals, and certain vitamins. Clearly, it's a good idea to get rid of them. In fact, the TLC diet includes few processed foods.

Here are some of the most common processed foods and where they hide:

- **Pantry:** These include boxed meals like macaroni and cheese; skillet dinners; prepared, packaged side dishes like prepared noodles, rice dishes, pastas, and potatoes; sugary cereals; high-sodium condiments; canned meals like soups, stews, and chili; sugary drinks like soda, energy drinks, and sports drinks; and refined breads, crackers, sugary ready-to-eat cereals, prepared rice, and pastas.

- **Refrigerator:** Here your biggest culprits are processed meats like hot dogs, bologna, sausage, bacon, deli meats, and ham. Whole-fat dairy is also high in saturated fat and can morph into many forms—chocolate milk, fruit yogurt, puddings, and cheesecake. Most whole-fat dairy is in the form of cheese, which can be found as an ingredient in many processed foods. Other full-fat dairy, like sour cream, creamy salad dressings, butter, cream cheese, and milk, appear here, too.
- **Freezer:** Frozen dinners and frozen pizza make up the bulk of frozen processed foods, but also beware of frozen appetizers, like mozzarella sticks, anything breaded and fried, chicken wings, mini pizzas, mini egg rolls, stuffed potatoes, and spinach dips. Frozen vegetables doused in butter or cheese sauce fall into this category as well.

Since most processed foods are made to last a long time, many can sit on your shelf for months or even years before they go bad. So what do you do with all the processed food you no longer want? You can donate it (if unopened) to a food pantry, give it away to someone you know who wants it, or simply keep it in a box in the basement (if they're pantry items) or on a special shelf in the refrigerator or freezer to be used gradually.

Get Rid of Fatty Snacks

We are a nation of snackers. According to the Institute of Food Technologists, snacking makes up about a quarter of the average American's caloric intake, making up what essentially is a fourth meal. So not only are we eating more calories at our regular meals, but we're also eating more calories throughout the day in the form of eating occasions. It's not unusual for some people to eat continuously, without ever giving themselves a chance to feel hungry.

GOTCHA!

On average, snacks eaten throughout the day total about 580 calories. That's equivalent to eating an extra fourth meal.

Unfortunately, most of these snacks are not good foods. Most are processed foods and sugary beverages—potato chips, nachos and dip, sugar-coated popcorn, candy bars or protein bars (which are often similar to candy bars), doughnuts, cookies, and cake.

These kinds of snacks are also more likely to contribute to your creeping weight gain over the years. That's what Harvard researchers found when they tracked the diets of more than 120,000 nonobese women. The main culprits: potato chips, potatoes (mainly french fries), sugar-sweetened beverages, red meat, and processed meats. Women who regularly ate these foods were more likely to gain weight over the years—on average, about 3.3 pounds every four years (more than 16 pounds in 20 years)—than those that didn't.

Not surprisingly, many people find that snacks are often the hardest to replace with healthy options. But this doesn't have to be the case. All it takes is a little planning to take control of your snacking behavior. To prevent yourself from rummaging around looking for food, plan your snacks like you plan your breakfast, lunch, and dinner. Plan for two snacks a day, and pick a specific time. Then make your snack a healthy one. (See "Load Up on Healthy Snacks" later in the chapter.)

Make Room for the Good Stuff

Now that you know what not to eat, it's time to talk about what to eat and what to stock your shelves with. Here's a quick rundown.

Fruits and vegetables. Clean out your vegetable and fruit bins, and make way for seasonal produce. Stock up on these good-for-you foods—but don't buy too much, or you'll end up throwing it out (see "Waste Not, Want Not" later in the chapter).

Small portions of lean meat, poultry, and fish. In the grocery store, I see many people load up on red meat and chicken. Instead, buy smaller portions so you can focus on vegetables instead of meat. If you do buy big packages, divvy them up in small packages of 2- to 3-ounce portions per person (about 6 to 8 ounces depending on the size of your family) as soon as you get home and freeze them.

Whole versus refined carbohydrates. This means having a pantry stocked with whole-wheat flour, brown rice, barley, quinoa, wild rice (and a variety of other kinds, like rice blends and black rice), and whole-grain breads and crackers. Stash your white sugar in the back of the cupboard or in the box of processed foods you stored away, and use less processed sweeteners, like honey, maple syrup, and evaporated cane sugar; if you do use them or other sugars, buy them in small jars or packages and use sparingly.

Stock up on beans. Dried beans last a long time on the shelves and come in a variety of colors, shapes, sizes, and flavors. Make beans ahead of time, then store in the refrigerator or freezer and pull them out when needed. Canned beans are another option, but beware of the sodium levels.

Low-fat or nonfat dairy. Always keep low-fat or nonfat dairy products like milk and yogurt in the refrigerator. There are also many high-quality reduced-fat cheeses on the market (Cabot Farms has an excellent low-fat cheddar—see cabotcreamery.com).

Plan for drinks. Think about what kinds of beverages you'll have in your house. Water is best; you might want to invest in a large pitcher and keep it filled in the refrigerator. But water isn't the only option. Make room for unsweetened tea or brewed tea, seltzer, coffee, or 100 percent fruit juices, but in small bottles. Remember, sugar calories from fruit juice can add up.

Load Up on Healthy Snacks

Once you have your pantry and your kitchen filled with healthful, good-for-you foods, finding healthful snacks is easy. But it still requires some planning. Fruit, for example, is more likely to be eaten if it's already cleaned, washed, and ready to go in the refrigerator (and placed up front). Since unhealthful snacking involves not only *what* we eat, but also *how much*, it's best to portion these foods ahead of time, in individual 100-calorie servings. Here are some ideas for healthy snacks:

- Fresh fruit
- Handful of nuts
- ½ cup nonfat, plain yogurt mixed with fresh fruit
- 3 cups air-popped popcorn, lightly seasoned, with no fat or little fat (margarine or oil)
- Cut-up celery or carrot sticks with dips like hummus
- Roasted and seasoned chickpeas
- Whole-wheat crackers with a small piece of low-fat cheese

Waste Not, Want Not

The biggest problem with switching to this new TLC lifestyle, and the biggest concern I hear from people, is that people buy these fresh fruits and vegetables with the best intentions but then don't use them and just end up throwing them out. As a nation, about 40 percent of the food we produce is wasted or thrown out. This includes food lost during farming, transportation, at supermarkets, and in restaurants.

> **HEALTHFUL LIVING**
>
> The average American throws out about 1¼ pounds of food each day.

Closer to home, the average American throws out more than one quarter of what's bought in the grocery store, amounting to about $2,200 worth of food each year for a family of four. Of this wasted food, vegetables are most likely to go in the trash. They're also the foods we should eat more of. Overbuying is perhaps the biggest reason these foods end up in the garbage, but it isn't the only reason. Here are a few ways to curb waste and eat healthfully without going overboard.

Plan Ahead

Buy just what you need at the grocery store. Make a list and stick to it. Once home, wash and prep your fresh fruits and vegetables as soon as you walk in the door. Although this takes more time up front, it will save you precious time later, when you want to use these foods. This will also increase your chance of using them.

If you're short on time, you may want to buy washed and bagged lettuce, spinach, and other greens. But remember, these have a shorter shelf life than whole produce and must be used in a day or two. If you don't think you're going to use them, don't buy them.

Make Smaller Portions

Many people on the TLC diet need to lose weight, which means they'll be eating less anyway. But even if you don't need to lose weight, it's important not to overeat. The best way to do this is to serve yourself smaller portions from the start. This way, you'll be less likely to overeat.

Retool Your Leftovers

If you do have leftovers, save them and eat them. Leftovers can be a lifesaver in terms of time and money management. Take soup, for example, which is good on several accounts. You can make soup ahead of time as a meal. It's a good way to use up bits and pieces of vegetables or meat in your refrigerator, and you can make it with homemade broths. When you make your own, you can generally keep it low in calories, high in fiber, and packed with colorful vegetables.

With a little bit of creativity and imagination, leftovers can make great lunches a day or two later. You can even transform some into salads or burritos. For example, Cuban Pork with Black Beans and Sweet Potatoes (recipe in Chapter 19) can morph into a salad over greens or can be rolled into a whole-wheat tortilla as a burrito.

Use Your Freezer

Clearing out all the high-fat, processed foods from your freezer means you'll have more room to freeze smaller portions or individual portions of homemade foods. Again, soups are a good example of this, but so is nearly any dish—roasted or cooked vegetables, whole grains, mixed dishes, and fresh or precooked and seasoned (by you) lean fish, chicken, or pork.

Having frozen meals ready to microwave will also prevent you from going out to dinner or grabbing fast food when you're hungry. And don't think of your freezer as just for storing already prepared completed meals. Ingredients also make great freezer companions.

Keep a stash of different types of unsweetened fruit in your freezer, and you can whip up a smoothie at a moment's notice. You can buy these fruits at the store or, in the case of blueberries or strawberries, wrap and freeze them straight from the farmers' market, store, or farm during peak season. This enables you to have fresh, peak-season fruit any time of the year.

Frozen vegetables, which are usually precooked by either boiling or roasting, are great go-to foods when you're looking for an interesting side dish or vegetable to round out a meal.

HEART-SMART HABITS

Learn to can. Although canning fruits usually requires a lot of sugar, canning vegetables doesn't. If you're not sure what to do, take a class and then start experimenting. This is another way to have whole, fresh, natural food all year long.

Have the Right Tools

Even though you have your kitchen well organized and well stocked with healthful, cholesterol-lowering, heart-healthy food, you're still not finished. Consider what you need to prepare this food. Having the right tools for the job is essential for creating delicious and nutritious meals you and your family will love.

Luckily, this doesn't need to cost a lot of money. You also don't need any fancy kitchen gadgets or gizmos. Just start with the basics, for now. If you're new to the culinary world, you may need to invest in some good-quality equipment for your kitchen. If you're not, it's still a good idea to re-evaluate your basic tools. Over the years, knives get dull, cutting boards stain, and pans chip and bowls crack. This may be a good time to reinvest in some new equipment.

A Set of Knives

Sharp knives are essential to any kitchen and make a huge difference when it comes to preparing and cooking healthful meals. They make slicing, dicing, and chopping faster, easier, and neater. That's because, instead of pushing your knife through the food, you are merely guiding it. While there are dozens of different types of knives on the market, designed according to their function, you really don't need that many, especially if you're just starting out.

If you have only two knives in your kitchen, I recommend a high-quality, stainless-steel chef's knife with an 8-inch blade and a good 3-inch paring knife. After that, you can acquire knives as you need them.

HEALTHFUL LIVING

The top three knife-making countries—Germany, Japan, and France—have a long heritage of crafting fine blades.

Remember, sharp knives won't stay sharp forever, particularly if you use them a lot. You may also want to invest in a knife sharpener or regularly get your knives sharpened by a professional. If you're cooking TLC food regularly, a good high-quality knife should last between six months and a year before it needs to be sharpened.

Pots and Pans

Pots and pans are staples in the kitchen, but before you go out and buy a big set, consider a few things first:

- **What you will be using them for:** If you don't like soup, don't buy a large stockpot. On the other hand, if stir-frying is your thing, be sure to have a large wok in your repertoire.

- **How much space you have:** Pots and pans take up a lot of space. Be sure you have enough room for what you want and need.
- **Ease of cleaning:** Do you want all your pans to go in the dishwasher, or are you okay washing them by hand? Some nonstick cookware cannot go in the dishwasher.
- **Budget and price:** Cookware sets can range from $50 to $2,000. Think about your budget before you go looking.

To start, I recommend getting a good set of nonstick pots and pans made of hard-anodized aluminum. Nonstick pots and pans require little or no fat in cooking and are better when cooking healthfully. Stainless-steel pots and pan are good conductors of heat but do require the use of fat to keep the food from sticking. They're also more expensive than nonstick brands.

Extras You Should Consider

Certainly, if you have the right pots, pans, and knives you're more than halfway to a well-stocked kitchen. You'll want a few more essential items, too:

- At least two sturdy plastic cutting boards—one for raw meat, fish, and poultry, and the other for everything else. Color coding helps. Wood is attractive but must be hand washed.
- A food scale and good set of measuring spoons and cups.
- A pizza or baking stone. Baking stones don't require any oil to prevent food from sticking. They also cook evenly in the oven. Every kitchen should have at least one stone, if not more.
- Serving spoons and utensils.
- A set of plastic storage containers for the freezer and the refrigerator.
- A zester and a vegetable peeler.

When it comes to eating a healthful diet, having the right tools and ingredients does more than make your life easier. It also fosters creativity and enjoyment, allowing you to appreciate and savor the wonderful healthful meals you will be producing.

The Least You Need to Know

- Getting rid of fatty, salty foods in your house is the first step to following the TLC diet. Not only will this help you stick to the plan, but it also will make room for more nutritious foods.
- Fill your TLC kitchen with healthy, nutritious foods, like fruits and vegetables, whole grains, lean meats, and low-fat or nonfat dairy.
- Stock your pantry and your refrigerator with healthful snacks like fruit, yogurt, raw vegetables, nuts, and beans, and stock your freezer with cooked or raw fruits and vegetables and homemade dishes.
- To save money and prevent waste, don't overbuy; instead, cook what you need and utilize leftovers. They can make your life a lot easier.
- To cook healthfully, you need the right tools. A well-stocked kitchen includes a variety of essential tools, including a good set of knives, pots and pans, and cutting boards.

Chapter

Smart Shopping

8

In This Chapter

- What to do before you go
- Tips for being a smart shopper
- Food labels interpreted
- Alternative markets for finding food

Now that you know what kinds of foods you'll be looking for and what kinds of foods you'll pass by, it's time to test your TLC smarts and take a trip to the grocery store. Some people dread shopping for groceries, but I find that most of those people don't know what kinds of food to buy and don't have a detailed plan or grocery list. You won't be one of those people.

After you read this chapter, you'll know where to find the kinds of foods you need, how to read nutrition and ingredient labels (and understand them!), and how to maneuver through the thousands of products now on the shelves. Be an informed shopper, and you won't be fooled by marketing hype or fancy packaging. You also won't be tricked into buying products that are touted as healthy but are not as good as they look.

Smart shoppers know that their first and most important step begins at home—before they even set foot in the store. Twenty minutes of prep time at home can save you hours of frustration at the store and at home. (Did you ever go to the store for one or two ingredients and come home an hour later with tons of groceries, but *not* the ingredient you went for?)

Follow the simple tips in this chapter, and your grocery trips will be relaxing, productive, fast, and efficient. And who knows? You may just enjoy them, too!

Do the Prep

Preparation is crucial for having a successful trip to the grocery store. And by *successful*, I mean buying healthful foods you like that are part of your TLC diet plan, buying everything you need to make complete meals for you and your family for at least several days, not overbuying, avoiding impulse purchases, and sticking to your budget. Without a plan before you go into the store, all these fall by the wayside.

Consider this scenario. You're driving home from work. You're tired and you're hungry, but you don't know what to make for dinner, so you stop at the grocery store to pick up a few things. At the store, you wander through the aisles choosing this and that. Sixty dollars later, you return home with bags of unhealthful foods—mainly snacks—and still nothing to make a balanced meal with. The end result? You order out for dinner.

HEALTHFUL LIVING

Last year, the first of the 76-million-strong baby boomers turned 65 years old. In supermarkets, their influence shows. Stores are offering more healthful food products, wider aisles, and lower shelves.

Many people complain that prep work before shopping, which includes planning menus, checking your pantry and refrigerator, and making a list, takes too much time and work. But consider how much time and money is wasted with the previous scenario. Then consider how much time and money good health is worth to you.

Another excuse I hear is, "I'll plan the menu and then no one will want to eat it, so why bother?" For this problem, I recommend planning only three or four menus at a time and creating meals that are flexible enough to be interchangeable. That way, if you or your family don't feel like eating one menu a certain day, you can offer the other menu. This is particularly easy with things you've already prepped, like a soup, which can be eaten in a few days, or a salad, which can be put together quickly but also has a few days' shelf life in the refrigerator.

Make a List and Check It Twice

The first thing to do before you go to the grocery store is plan the foods you want to eat. How many days you plan your menu for depends on what kind of shopper you are. Some people hate grocery shopping and go only once a month. For them, menu planning probably involves two or three weeks' worth of meals, taking into account eating leftover meals and going out to dinner. On the other extreme are people who go shopping every day—this is not a good practice. According to a 2008 study by the Marketing Science Institute, people who take "quick trips" to the grocery store end up buying 54 percent more food than they planned.

On average, however, most people make one big trip to the grocery store every week or so. This could be to a traditional supermarket, a big warehouse or club store, a superstore, or any combination of these. For example, during the summer, I go to a farmers' market once a week and a traditional supermarket once every two weeks, but during the winter, this pattern flip-flops.

For most people, making up about five or six days of menus, with an extra day for leftovers or a grab-'n'-go day (in my house, that means a smoothie or yogurt-and-fruit dinner once in a while), is probably enough. When planning your menus, be sure to focus on fresh, wholesome, natural foods and minimize foods high in saturated fat, like cheese and meat. Also keep in mind what seasonal ingredients are available. See Chapter 10 for menu ideas.

HEALTHFUL LIVING

According to the Food Marketing Institute, in 2012, the average consumer made 2.2 trips to the supermarket per week and spent $26.78 per each customer transaction.

When you've got your menu down, you need to create a second list on a separate piece of paper. List all the ingredients you need for the menus you wrote for the week. Check the list against your pantry, fridge, and freezer to make sure you don't buy what you already have. It's also a good idea to check this list against store sales flyers and any coupons you may have.

Be sure to include staples, which may not be on your menu but which you always keep a supply in the house. This could be oatmeal; vegetable oil; any spices; low-fat, low-sodium deli meats; low-fat yogurt; whole-wheat, high-fiber breads and crackers; tuna; hummus; roasted red peppers in a jar; nonfat milk, soy milk, or almond milk; nuts; and anything else you eat on a regular basis. Some people factor in a cushion (usually based on a dollar amount) for foods they may not plan for—planned impulse purchases. This is okay as long as these purchases are healthful foods that fit into the TLC diet.

You may also want to keep a running list of low-fat, low-sodium foods and the brands you like. This is particularly helpful when brands among products vary greatly, like in cereals or soups.

To make things go smoother and faster in the store, organize your list. You can do this in two ways. First, if you know the store well, you can organize the list by aisle. Otherwise, I recommend just grouping like foods together, such as all dairy, all meats, all canned goods, and so on.

This takes some time and is usually best done on a weekend or day when you've planned a shopping trip. But what happens if you want to stop at the grocery store after work? You can still avoid the unhealthful traps of impulse purchases and overspending mentioned earlier. Before you enter the store, simply spend a few minutes in the car writing a list of exactly what you plan to eat tonight (and tomorrow, if possible), along with the ingredients you need to buy to make it.

Although this quick method doesn't guarantee you won't buy things you already have at home, it will save you from making less nutritious impulse purchases, not to mention save you from wasting time and money.

Eat Before You Go

The last two things you have to remember are just as important as writing a list:

- Don't go grocery shopping hungry.
- Don't bring children or spouses.

Everyone knows a hungry shopper buys more at the store. To prevent your stomach from making purchasing decisions for you, eat before you go, or keep a stash of dried fruit, nuts, and water (if you can) in the car. This will take the edge off your hunger and help you be a better shopper.

Children and spouses are more likely to persuade you to buy things that are not on your list. Young children especially are prone to food marketers' ploys for buying sugary cereals and other unhealthful snacks. Do yourself a favor and leave the spouse and kids or grandkids at home. If you can't, set some rules for what your kids can and cannot buy before entering the store. Then use that time to teach your kids how to make smart food choices.

At the Store

Once you're at the store, don't be overwhelmed by its size or flashy marketing hype. Traditional supermarkets can carry as many as 60,000 SKU (stock-keeping units) products on their shelves, all vying for your attention and dollars. Many now offer a service deli, service bakery, and pharmacy, too.

Remember, supermarkets are designed to sell products, and they thrive on impulse purchases. They also thrive on selling highly processed, fatty, sugary foods, so keep that in mind when you wheel your cart down the aisles. Be confident knowing you are armed with your health-oriented grocery list, and stick to it.

HEART-SMART HABITS

Usually the most expensive and most highly processed (read: high-calorie, high-fat, and high-salt) products are located on grocery store shelves at eye level. Food manufacturers pay a premium for this space. Check the upper and lower shelves, and you're likely to find better deals for both your pocketbook and your health.

Hit the Produce Section

Most grocery stores are planned so that you enter the produce aisle first, for two main reasons. First it creates a positive image of fresh, healthful food. Second, it encourages impulse purchases because of the many sale items listed. Since the TLC diet emphasizes vegetables and fruits as a large part of your diet, loading up on produce is a good idea—but beware of overbuying. Stick to your list. Other tips to keep in mind:

- Buy a wide variety of fruits and vegetables in an array of different colors.
- Buy produce in season and locally grown, if possible. This is usually cheaper and of peak quality.
- Look for quality. Fresh fruits and vegetables are always better than processed ones, but if something doesn't look good, don't buy it. Remember, frozen vegetables and fruits are another option and at times may be a better choice (and of better quality) than fresh produce.
- Buy precut or bagged produce only if you're going to use it right away. These products have a much shorter shelf life than fresh produce. Still, buying bagged or precut vegetables is a great time saver if you're in a rush. Be sure to check the best-used-by date, which signifies peak quality. Sometimes it's okay to use after this date, but taste and texture may be slightly altered.

Cruise the Inner Aisles

Most of the foods sold in the inner aisles of the grocery store are not the types of food you want to be eating on the TLC diet. Thus, plan on a quick foray through these aisles and plan on buying only the items you have on your list. Here are some of the heart-healthy foods you're likely to find there:

- Whole grains, like oatmeal, barley, brown rice, some whole-grain cereals, pastas, crackers, and flours.
- Vegetable oils, such as corn, canola, olive, or soybean oil.
- Dried herbs and spices.
- Vinegars, like balsamic, wine, white, and apple cider.
- Dark chocolate.
- Dried beans, peas and legumes.
- Snacks—but choose snacks low in sodium and fat, with no added sugar. Look for high-fiber options, in single servings or 100-calorie serving packages.
- Nuts, seeds, and nut butters.
- Unsweetened drinks, like water and tea.
- Certain condiments, such as mustard, olives, and capers. Try to choose food that is as close to its natural state as possible.
- Some canned goods.

Let me say a word about canned foods. Canned foods are okay on occasion; however, they should not be a regular part of your diet, for several reasons. Many canned vegetable products and brined foods are high in sodium, which is not good for your heart or your blood pressure. In fact, even low-sodium canned products (this is true for broths) may still be considered a high-sodium food. No-salt-added canned foods are a good option, but they are not always easy to find. Canned fruit is more likely to be packed in sugary syrup or even fruit juice, which is also high in sugar.

HEART-SMART HABITS

Visit the bulk bins. Here you can often find nuts, dried fruits, and sometimes whole grains at a much lower price.

Finally, canned foods contain BPA (bisphenol A). BPA is a compound that is used in plastics to line the inside of cans, the coating on cash register receipts, and hundreds of other things. In the body, it disrupts hormones and is particularly harmful for pregnant women and young children. Recently, though, researchers have linked BPA to heart disease. In the latest study, completed in 2012 in England, researchers looked at urine samples of more than 1,500 adults during a 10-year period. The people who developed heart disease had higher concentrations of BPA in their blood at the start of this period, compared to those who stayed free of heart disease. While we still don't know the extent to which BPA increases risk, this study shows it may be a major contributor to heart disease risk.

To reduce your exposure to BPA, look for tomatoes, tuna, beans, and other products in a carton, pouch, or jar or in the freezer section. Or look for companies that use BPA-free cans. One company known for their BPA-free cans is Eden Organic. However, not all organic foods are BPA free; in fact, most aren't.

Walk the Perimeter

Most of the more healthful products are located around the outside of the store. This includes fresh meat, fish, and poultry; low-fat dairy; eggs; whole-grain breads (sometimes); juices; and frozen foods. Since these foods need to be kept cold, try to make them last on your list. On the other hand, buying them early means you'll be spending less time grocery shopping.

GOTCHA!

Stay away from endcaps. These are the special promotions at the front or back of every aisle. They are most likely to be an impulse purchase and often include less-than-healthful foods.

Learn Label Lingo

Reading labels is essential for choosing the right foods—healthful foods low in fat, calories, cholesterol, sodium, and sugar. You also want foods high in fiber and vitamins and minerals. Produce, of course, needs no explanation, but for nearly everything else, it's imperative that you read both the nutrition facts panel and the ingredient list.

The Nutrition Facts Panel

The nutrition facts panel gives you a quick nutritional snapshot of the food. All the nutrients are listed in gram or milligram amounts except for the vitamins, which are listed as percentages of what we need (daily values). By law, the nutrition label has to list 10 nutrients: total fat, saturated fat, trans fats, cholesterol, sodium, total carbohydrates, dietary fiber, sugars, and protein. Plus, it must list four vitamins and minerals: vitamin A, C, calcium, and iron. Manufacturers have the option to add more information, but they cannot get away with less, unless the food does not contain significant amounts of that nutrient.

The more you read labels, the better you'll get at deciphering them—and the more you'll use them to make good choices. Here's what you need to look at.

Serving size and servings per container. The serving size is based on standard measures, like cups or pieces. Similar foods usually have similar serving sizes so you can compare, but not always (for example, serving sizes for cereal can range from $\frac{1}{2}$ cup, to $\frac{1}{3}$ cup, to 1 cup or more).

Sometimes a package you expect to be one serving is actually two servings, such as with beverages or frozen meals. So always check the servings per container and compare that to what you think you will actually eat. If you eat two servings of a food, remember to double all the nutrition facts panel numbers.

Calories per serving and calories of fat per serving. This shows you how many calories are in one serving of food and how many calories come from fat.

Percent daily values. Percent daily value shows you how much of a specific nutrient one serving has as a percentage of the entire day, based on a 2,000-calorie diet. For example, a product with 10 grams of total fat has a daily value of 15 percent. That means this product would be 15 percent of your total intake of fat for the entire day based on a 2,000-calorie diet. Use these numbers as a guide to see if a product is high or low in something—and remember, if you take in fewer than 2,000 calories, these percentages would be higher.

Nutrients to Watch Out For

The nutrients you want to keep track of are total fat, saturated fat, trans fats, cholesterol, and sodium. Since most of the foods you look at will be either parts of a meal (ingredients) or one meal, you want these numbers to be no more than a third (preferably less) of your max. You also have to keep in mind what you will be eating for the rest of the day.

For saturated fats, you probably want to keep this number around 1 to 2 grams—no more than 3 grams per serving. Trans fats should be as close to 0 as possible, cholesterol should stay under 200 milligrams, and sodium should be about 150 to 250 milligrams or less.

Also pay attention to sugar intake. The sugars on labels include *both* natural sugars and added sugars. This makes a difference. Natural sugars found in dried fruit or dairy products also come packaged with other healthful nutrients. Added sugars are simply sugar. The only way you can tell whether a food has added sugars is to read the ingredient label (I talk about that next). Generally, however, you want to keep those sugar numbers low, natural or not. If it is simply added sugar, keep those numbers low—around 10 grams of sugar per 100-gram serving (you can figure out gram amounts from the serving size).

Nutrients to Get More Of

These are the nutrients you want to increase in your diet. They include fiber and the vitamins and minerals. Try to choose foods that provide 4 to 5 grams of fiber per serving and vitamin levels above 15 percent.

HEALTHFUL LIVING

To be a good source of a nutrient, a food must contain 10 to 19 percent of the daily value. An excellent source has 20 percent or more of the daily value. For vitamins and minerals, the daily value is the same as the recommended dietary allowance (RDA).

Ingredient Buzzwords

On any healthful diet, reading ingredient labels as well as nutrition facts panels is essential. By law, all packaged food sold in retail must list all the foods contained in that product. However, if an item contains less than .5 gram per serving of a particular ingredient, the manufacturer can list it as being 0 on the nutrition facts panel. For this reason, it's always important to check ingredient lists against nutrition facts labels, particularly for trans fats, which shows up on ingredient lists as partially hydrogenated fat.

Ingredients are always listed in descending order by weight. Thus, the first ingredient is always what the food contains the most of. As a general rule, the shorter the list, the better, and the more whole natural ingredients (and words you can pronounce), the better.

Besides fat, there are a few other things to look for on ingredient lists, like artificial sweeteners. Keep this tip in mind: artificial sweeteners are usually last on the list, so if you don't read through, you can easily miss them. (My husband is notorious for doing this.) Why? Artificial sweeteners are hundreds of times sweeter than natural sweeteners, so you need only a miniscule amount to sweeten a food. Thus, the amount of the ingredient by weight is very low. The same holds true for monosodium glutamate, which is something to note if you are sensitive to it or are watching your salt.

Beware of added sugars and sweeteners. These are usually listed separately on the ingredient list, but they can really add up.

GOTCHA!

To downplay how much sugar a specific food actually contains, many food manufacturers list sugars separately throughout the ingredient list. In one popular cereal, sugar was listed 12 times in the ingredient label in 8 different forms.

All of these terms are simply another way of saying sugar:

Agave nectar
Beet sugar
Brown rice syrup
Brown sugar
Cane sugar
Corn syrup
Corn syrup solids
Dextrin
Dextrose
Evaporated cane juice
Fructose
Fructose sweetener
High-fructose corn syrup
Honey
Invert sugar
Liquid fructose
Maltodextrin
Molasses
Raw sugar
Sorghum syrup
Sucrose
Turbinado sugar
White sugar

Beware of Banners

Many food manufacturers make claims regarding the nutrient content of their products. Unfortunately, not all foods that make nutrient content claims are good choices for the TLC diet. In fact, many are not. Nevertheless, the Food and Drug Administration regulates these claims with strict definitions:

Calorie free: Fewer than 5 calories per serving

Low calorie: 40 or fewer calories per serving

Cholesterol free: Less than 2 milligrams of cholesterol and less than 2 milligrams of saturated fat

Low cholesterol: 20 milligrams of cholesterol or less, and less than 2 milligrams of saturated fat

Reduced cholesterol: At least 25 percent less cholesterol than the regular product and less than 2 milligrams of saturated fat

Fat free, saturated fat free, or trans fat free: Less than .5 gram of fat, saturated fat, or trans fat

Low fat: 3 grams of fat or less

Low saturated fat: 1 gram of saturated fat or less, with no more than 15 percent of calories coming from saturated fat

Reduced fat or less fat: At least 25 percent less fat than the original version

High fiber: 5 grams or more of fiber per serving

Good source of fiber: 2.5 to 4.9 grams of fiber per serving

Lean: Less than 10 grams of fat, 4.5 grams of saturated fat, and 95 milligrams of cholesterol

Extra lean: Less than 5 grams of fat, 2 grams of saturated fat, and 95 milligrams of cholesterol

Light (lite): One third fewer calories than the regular product, or no more than half the fat of the regular product, or no more than half the sodium of the regular product

Sodium free or salt free: Less than 5 milligrams of sodium and no sodium chloride in the ingredients

Low sodium: 140 mg of sodium or less per serving

Reduced or less sodium: At least 25 percent less sodium than the regular product

Very low sodium: 35 milligrams of sodium or less

Sugar free: Less than .5 gram of sugar

Reduced sugar: At least 25 percent less sugar than the regular product

GOTCHA!

Beware of products labeled "reduced sugar," "less sugar," or "lite." More often than not, they contain artificial sweeteners and may even taste sweeter than their regular sugar counterparts.

Shop Local Farmers' Markets

While the majority of our population still buys their food from conventional supermarkets, more people are turning to alternative sources, particularly when searching for healthful food. This has led to a booming farmers' market business across the country. At farmers' markets, farmers sell their produce directly to the consumer.

Although prices are not necessarily lower—and often, in fact, may be higher—the quality is usually head and shoulders above what you would find at your traditional supermarket. Here you can be assured that you're getting the freshest, best-tasting, and most nutritious product you can (most produce was picked within 24 hours). So if you're looking for unbeatable seasonal produce, farmers' markets are a good bet.

Other places to find high-quality fresh, healthful food are specialty stores like Whole Foods and other organic markets, buying clubs, farm stores, community-supported agriculture (CSA) groups, and even your own backyard vegetable garden.

Finding good-for-you food that's nutritious and delicious isn't as hard as you think if you just look for it. While it does take some practice, once you get used to shopping this way, you'll find healthful offerings just about everywhere you go.

The Least You Need to Know

- The best way to navigate your grocery store for healthful foods is to make a list of what you want to buy and stick to it.
- Supermarkets are designed to sell products and thrive on impulse purchases. Don't be tricked into buying unhealthful foods you don't need.

- Most of your purchases should be foods found around the perimeter of the store, like produce; low-fat dairy; fresh lean meat, chicken, or fish; juices; and whole grains.
- To make good choices, it's crucial to read both nutrition labels and ingredient labels and then compare the two.
- When looking for healthful food, keep in mind farmers' markets and specialty stores in addition to the healthy sections of conventional grocery stores.

Chapter 9

Picking the Best Proteins

In This Chapter

- Choosing leaner red meat
- How much chicken and poultry is enough?
- Finding the right fish for you
- Plants have protein, too

You don't have to give up red meat on the TLC diet, nor do you have to live on chicken breasts. You will, however, probably have to reevaluate the way you think about meat and protein in general. Big slabs of steak, half-pound hamburgers, and buckets of fried chicken or fried fish are no longer part of your meal plan. These foods are not good for your health. They are also bad for the environment and the land.

Your meals will not center on meat, chicken, or even fish, but rather will emphasize produce like vegetables, fruits, and legumes. You will also be eating two or three vegetarian or vegan meals a week. Not only will this save you money, but you'll be right on track with today's current dietary trends. Vegetarian entrées have become a hot trend on restaurant menus, and many consumers, young and old, now regularly eat vegetarian meals even though they're not vegetarian. Health, taste, and concern for the environment are the top three reasons for this, but there are also social, political, and religious reasons. To get you started thinking meatless, Chapter 20 features only vegetarian and vegan recipes.

When you do choose meat, poultry, or fish, you want to choose the option that is best for your health, your budget, and your cooking style. On the TLC diet, you'll be looking for lean cuts of beef, pork, or lamb; low-fat chicken; and, surprisingly, fatty fish (lean fish is good, too). In this chapter, I show you what kinds of protein you should and should not eat and explain why. I also put to rest some concerns you may have about getting enough protein. This is a problem few Americans face, but many people still worry about it. In fact, even if you don't eat any meat, fish, or chicken, protein is generally not an issue. Not convinced? Read on.

Can I Eat Red Meat?

Many people who have had a heart attack or have high cholesterol automatically assume that they need to give up red meat. That's not true. Yes, you can eat red meat on the TLC diet. You just need to eat the right kind of red meat (lean cuts) and the right amount (2 to 3 ounces). All kinds of meat are naturally high in saturated fat and cholesterol. But some cuts are definitely better than others.

Top Lean Choices

The fat in red meat is basically found in two places. The first place is around the outside of the meat muscle. This is called the external fat, and it is the visible white fat you see around the meat. Visible fat is easy to spot and easy to remove. Depending on your butcher, you can have this fat trimmed anywhere from 1 inch to $\frac{1}{8}$ inch. You want to remove all external fat.

The second type of fat is the fat in between the muscle fibers inside the meat. This is called marbling, and it's what gives meat it's tender, melt-in-your mouth quality. But it's also what makes meat so high in fat, especially saturated fat. Marbling looks like tiny white streaks scattered throughout the meat. The cut of meat most known for its extensive marbling is filet mignon. A petite $3\frac{1}{2}$-ounce portion trimmed of all external fat has 231 calories, 12 grams of fat, 5 grams of saturated fat, and 90 milligrams of cholesterol. Compare this to a $3\frac{1}{2}$-ounce serving of a top round steak, with 186 calories, 5.6 grams of total fat, 2 grams of saturated fat, and 84 milligrams of cholesterol. The top round steak contains less than half the fat and saturated fat as the filet mignon, and it costs less, too.

The USDA grades meat according to quality. Quality is based on fat content and age of the animal, among other factors. Prime is the highest quality and also the fattiest cuts. Most of these cuts end up in food service. Next come Choice and Select. This is what you're most likely to see in retail stores. When it comes to choosing lean cuts, you want to go for the Select.

GOTCHA!

Beware of processed meats like bologna, sausage, salami, and hot dogs. Even those labeled as reduced fat or reduced sodium are still generally high in fat, saturated fat, and sodium.

When it comes to choosing lean cuts of red meat, like beef, lamb, and pork, you want to look for the words *round* and *loin*. In beef, these are round, chuck, sirloin, and loin cuts. In pork, these are tenderloin and loin chop; in lamb, they're the leg, arm, and loin. Cuts with the term *extra lean* are also good choices.

Even when you do choose lean cuts, remember to watch portion sizes. On the TLC diet, you want a total of only 5 ounces or less of meat, poultry, or fish a day. That means a serving would most likely be 2 to 3 ounces, at most. If you want an idea of how much that is, look at the recipes in Chapters 16, 18, and 19. All the protein choices contain 3 ounces or less.

Go for Grass-Fed

Typical commercial livestock is raised on mainly corn, usually combined with soybeans, cottonseed meal, and hay. Feeding cows and pigs this way makes them gain weight quickly. But along with muscle, these animals also put on more fat.

Consequently, grass-fed beef is leaner than traditionally raised beef. The meat itself also has a different nutritional composition. Compared to conventional beef, grass-fed meat is lower in saturated fat and higher in omega-3 fatty acids, beta-carotene (vitamin A), and conjugated linoleic acid (CLA). CLA is associated with lower heart disease and cancer risk. Unlike conventional beef, grass-fed beef also contains vitamin E, an antioxidant that has heart-protective qualities. And because grass-fed cows tend to be healthier than conventional cows, they are less likely to be given antibiotics and growth hormones.

But before you run to the store to stock up on grass-fed beef, keep this in mind: grass-fed beef tastes different than conventional beef. Corn-fed beef tends to be mild in flavor; grass-fed beef is earthier and more robust, with a more distinct taste. It's also more expensive than conventional beef and could easily run twice the price.

GOTCHA!

Grass-fed beef that's corn finished means the animal is usually given corn during the last few months of its life. Although this is a short period, it is enough to change the fatty acid composition of the meat to be more like conventional beef, negating any health benefits.

Try Bison and Venison

If you have the opportunity to eat bison or venison, do it. Game meat is leaner and healthier for you than commercially raised livestock. That's because these animals eat plants, seeds, and nuts that Mother Nature provides. They also are more active than domestically raised animals and so have less fat. Lastly, there is a genetic difference in the meat from rabbit, deer, moose, or elk, making it nutritionally different from beef (usually in a more positive way).

Take bison or buffalo, for example. A surge in demand has created a booming commercial industry for this breed. Although still considered "wild," many of these animals are now corn fed. Though grass-fed bison is still better than corn-fed bison, both are lower in fat and calories than most cuts of beef and chicken. That's because, genetically, bison contain no marbling, so the meat is leaner than beef. To get the real deal, look for grass-fed bison at local farmers' markets and online (bison is raised in every state of the union). Grass-fed bison has all the benefits of grass-fed cows and more.

Adapting Your Cooking Style

If you're not used to cooking lean meat, switching to leaner cuts may take some getting used to in the kitchen. Because they contain less fat, leaner cuts cook more quickly, so it's easy to overcook them. Once overcooked, they get dry, tough, and stringy. Consequently, many lean cuts are best served rare.

How you cook them—broil, grill, stew, or braise—depends on the cut of meat and the way you want to prepare it. In general, the best rule of thumb is "low and slow." Here are a few other tips that work well with lean cuts:

- Season well with herbs and spices.
- Use marinades to keep the meat moist and add flavor.
- Cook meat on a rack so the fat and juices can drip down and you can drain them off.
- Cook soups and stews the night before, then refrigerate them and skim off the fat before reheating.
- For tougher cuts of meat, consider cutting them in small strips for fajitas or a stir-fry. They'll cook quickly and be more tender.

What about organ meats like liver, sweetbreads, tongue, and kidneys? Although they're not high in fat, these foods are generally high in cholesterol. If you do eat them, consider them a special treat and splurge only about once a month.

Birds of a Feather

Chicken is certainly the most popular protein on most cholesterol-lowering diets, followed by turkey. In fact, turkey has grown from being a once-a-year food to an everyday meal (mostly in the form of sandwiches) for many people. Not surprisingly, turkey consumption has more than doubled in the last 25 years.

Both turkey and chicken can be good choices on the TLC diet plan because they are low in fat and saturated fat. Most of the fat in chicken is located under the skin, so if you remove the skin, you remove the fat. Some people remove the skin before they cook it; others remove it afterward. Either way is fine. Removing the chicken skin after you cook it prevents the chicken breast from drying out during cooking. But it also makes it harder for you to resist eating. If you are preparing the chicken with any kind of special seasoning or breading, it's best to take off the skin before you fix it; this way, the meat will absorb the seasoning, not the skin.

Keep in mind, too, that chicken also contains yellow fat deposits, usually around the thigh and sometimes the breast. You can easily remove these when you clean the chicken.

Turkey is sold in parts, and like chicken, the white meat is leaner than the dark (see the following section). You can now buy turkey breasts all year long. One tip is to bake a turkey breast, slice it thinly, and place it in small packages for freezing. Then you can pull it out and use it for sandwiches later.

Canned meat like white meat chicken is another option, but also something to watch out for. Although it is low in fat and inexpensive, it is high in sodium. To lower the sodium, check different brands (sodium levels vary) and be sure to rinse the meat before eating.

White Meat vs. Dark Meat

Chicken white meat is lean. Without the skin, one $3\frac{1}{2}$-ounce serving has only about 165 calories, 3.6 grams total fat, 1 gram saturated fat, and 85 milligrams cholesterol. The same amount of dark meat, on the other hand, has 205 calories, 10 grams total fat, 2.6 grams saturated fat, and 93 milligrams cholesterol.

That's not to say that you can't ever eat dark meat, but be aware that white meat should be your first choice. Avoid chicken wings, which are naturally high in fat and skin, and are usually made doubly worse by deep-fat frying.

And although most people are familiar with chicken in its fried form, you can prepare it in many more healthful ways, including grilling, broiling, baking, sautéing, stir-frying, oven-frying, poaching, and braising. Because it has a mild, neutral flavor, chicken pairs well with almost any seasoning or spice blend.

Ground Meat

Ground turkey and chicken are another popular pick, but read the label before you buy. Some ground turkey or chicken has skin and fat ground up; other packages are pure meat. The only way to tell is to look at the label. Packages with only ground meat will read "ground turkey breast" or "ground chicken breast." Ground meat is also often labeled by percent fat by weight, usually as percent lean or percent fat. You want to choose the leanest one, such as 95 percent lean or 5 percent fat.

Another option is to check the nutrition label. As of March 2012, all fresh meat products, including ground chicken, turkey, beef, and pork, are required to have a nutrition label. The label is based on a 4-ounce raw portion, which translates into 3 ounces cooked. It lists fat, saturated fat, cholesterol, and other required nutrients, making it easy to compare products and choose more healthful options.

Duck and Goose

Unlike red meat, the majority of fat located on ducks and geese is underneath the skin. Consequently, if you remove the skin and the thick layer of fat beneath it, you are removing much of the fat. Nevertheless, goose and duck meat is still pretty fatty, making it more of a once-in-a-while treat than a regular offering. One $3\frac{1}{2}$-ounce portion of duck or goose meat (goose is slightly fattier) has roughly 4 grams of saturated fat, has 11 to 12 grams of total fat, and supplies 200 to 238 calories.

From the Sea

Fish and seafood are an excellent source of high-quality protein. They are also our best supply of the heart-protective omega-3 fatty acids, EPA (eicosapentaenoic acid), and DHA (docosahexaenoic acid). DHA and EPA are mainly found in fatty fish, but lean fish have benefits, too. On the TLC diet, you should be eating fatty fish at least two times a week and consuming other varieties another one or two times, for a total of about four or more meals a week (about 8 to 12 ounces a week or more).

Canned fish or fish sold in a pouch (like tuna or salmon) is also a good choice, particularly if you are on a budget, as it is an inexpensive, high-quality lean protein. Look for low-sodium brands.

HEART-SMART HABITS

Another type of omega-3 fatty acid, ALA (alpha-linolenic acid), is found only in plant foods like tofu, soybeans, flaxseeds, and walnuts. ALA can be converted to DHA and EPA in small amounts. In several studies, ALA-rich foods have been found to reduce the risk of heart disease. Whether you have heart disease or want to prevent it, it's a good idea to include these foods in your diet on a regular basis.

If you're concerned about mercury, don't worry. Most commercial seafood contains only small amounts of this pollutant. If you stay away from shark, swordfish, tilefish, and king mackerel, and eat a variety of seafood, you should be fine. In fact, study after study has shown that the benefit of eating seafood for your health far outweighs the small risk from low doses of mercury.

Best Bets for Finfish

Finfish fall into two camps: lean fish and oily fish. Incorporate a mix of both types of seafood in your diet, for the sake of variety as well as health. Lean fin fish include tilapia, cod, pollock, flounder or sole, rockfish, catfish, and orange roughy, to name a few. Because they're low in omega-3 fatty acids, lean fish don't have the same cardiac benefits as fatty fish, but they do offer many other advantages. They're high in protein and important vitamins and minerals, especially iodine, selenium, and potassium. They can also be a boon for people looking to lose weight or manage weight loss. Finally, a recent study showed that eating lean fish four times a week reduced blood pressure in coronary heart disease subjects.

Oily or fatty fish tend to be of the cold water variety because fish living in this environment produce more fat for insulation. These are salmon, barramundi, rainbow trout, herring, fresh tuna, mackerel, sardines, and anchovies. How much omega-3 fatty acids a fish has depends on the type of fish and how it was raised or lived. For example, in general, wild salmon has more omega-3 fatty acids than farmed salmon, even though farmed salmon may be fattier. For more information on seafood, check out aboutseafood.com.

What About Shellfish?

Shellfish include mollusks like crabs, oysters, scallops, and mussels, and crustaceans like crab, shrimp, and lobster. These foods have a reputation for being high in cholesterol yet low in fat, saturated fat, and calories. Most fall in the range of 80 to 95 milligrams of cholesterol per 3-ounce portion, with the exception of shrimp, which contains about twice that amount, 170 milligrams of cholesterol. Fresh shrimp also has another drawback: depending on how it's treated, it can be high in sodium. For this reason, I have not included any shrimp recipes in this book.

What is the bottom line when it comes to shellfish? Eat it occasionally but not on a regular basis. Also keep in mind that cholesterol content varies depending on the shellfish—for instance, mussels and clams are usually lower in cholesterol than squid and oysters.

Plants Have Protein, Too

When people decrease the meat, poultry, and fish in their diet, they often feel like they're shortchanging themselves on protein. But that's not the case. In the typical American diet, most people get more protein than they need, and excess protein ends up being converted to fat. According to the most recent National Health and Nutrition Examination Survey (2005–2006), the average male takes in more than 100 grams of protein a day, and women average about 70. That's twice as much as what health experts say we need.

The U.S. recommended dietary allowances suggests .8 gram of protein per kilogram (kg) body weight. To get your weight in kilograms, divide your weight in pounds by 2.2. For a 165-pound person, that equals about 75 kilograms. Multiply that by .8, and you have a daily protein intake of about 60 grams. As you increase physical activity, protein needs increase, but the jump is still not that much. (Healthy active adults generally up their protein intake to 1.2 grams per kilogram of body weight. For a 165-pound person, that's 90 grams—still below average for male intakes.)

If your protein intake is low, eating the TLC way can get you on track for getting the proper amount (10 to 25 percent of calories daily).

So where does our protein come from? While the most concentrated and common sources of protein in the American diet are meat, chicken, fish, and cheese—1 ounce of these foods contains about 7 grams of protein—these are not the only places we get protein. This nutrient is also found in bread, whole grains, vegetables, and fruits (yes, fruits), but in smaller amounts (most range from 1 to 5 grams per serving). In the plant world, the protein powerhouses are beans, soybeans, quinoa, and nut butters, like peanut butter—these foods average about 7 or 8 grams protein per serving.

HEART-SMART HABITS

One cup of red beans, combined with 1 cup of brown rice and $\frac{1}{2}$ cup tomato sauce, supplies 22 grams of protein, the equivalent of about 3 ounces of steak.

Unlike animal protein, plant protein is not complete. Protein is made up of amino acids. We need 20 amino acids from our diet. These are called essential amino acids. If a protein has all 20 amino acids, it is considered complete. If it is lacking even one amino acid, it is incomplete. This means the food must be combined with another food high in the missing amino acid. All animal proteins are complete; nearly all plant proteins are incomplete, with two exceptions: soybeans and quinoa. That's not a problem, however: combined, the two main food groups—legumes and whole grains—provide complete proteins. Don't worry about combining them in meals, either—if you're following a plant-based diet, you'll automatically eat enough.

People who eat a completely plant-based diet, such as vegans, usually have no problem getting enough protein. On the TLC diet, you'll be focusing on vegetable proteins rather than animal ones. Vegetable proteins are lower in saturated fat than animal proteins and also contain no cholesterol. Furthermore, research shows that people who eat vegetable proteins and fats have lower rates of heart disease than people who eat animal-based proteins and fats.

Lean meat, fish, or chicken can easily fit into the TLC diet plan, as long as you eat it in small amounts. Eventually, as you learn to love vegetables, whole grains, and beans, you won't even miss the meat.

The Least You Need to Know

- Red meat like beef, pork, and lamb can fit into the TLC diet plan as long as you keep portions small (between 2 and 3 ounces) and choose lean cuts, like sirloin or round.
- Choose the white meat of chicken or turkey over dark meat, and remove the skin to reduce saturated fat.
- To protect your heart and your health, plan on two or three meals each week that include fatty fish, like salmon or sardines.
- When planning vegetarian meals, focus on plant proteins like beans, soy (tofu), and quinoa in place of animal proteins.

Lifestyle Secrets to Success

Part 3

The TLC diet is more than just an eating plan—it's a lifestyle. You'll change not only what you eat, but also when and how you eat. In this part, you learn how to create healthful menus using my seven-day menu plan as a guide, which offers different calorie levels so you can make adjustments. Learning a new approach to food means breaking old, bad habits and creating good, new ones to take their place. I give you strategies for overcoming some of the problems people face when making changes to their diet. When it comes to following the TLC diet, the first step involves commitment to yourself and your loved ones. This part will keep you motivated and inspired to do your best. Finally, I give you suggestions on what to do if your diet is not working and your numbers aren't coming down as fast as you want.

Menus for Losing Weight

Chapter 10

In This Chapter

- Basic guidelines for losing weight
- Foods to mix and match
- Coming up with a plan that works for you
- Sample daily menus for 1,200, 1,500, 1,800, and 2,000 calories

As you know from previous chapters, being overweight is a major risk factor for developing heart disease. It also increases your risk of other health problems, like diabetes. Where you put on the weight makes a difference, too: people who have bigger bellies have a much higher risk of having heart disease than those who have extra weight around the hips and thighs.

Although not everyone who has high cholesterol is overweight, excess weight can cause problems. It may result in more fat circulating in the blood, leading to higher-than-normal levels of blood cholesterol and triglycerides. There's also a good chance you'll have high blood pressure and high blood sugar. The good news is, it doesn't take much to turn things around. Losing as little as 10 to 15 pounds or 5 to 10 percent of your body weight can significantly improve blood lipid levels and lower both blood pressure and blood sugar levels.

Many people on the TLC diet lose weight without even trying. Mostly, that's because you're cutting out high-calorie junk food and replacing it with low-fat, healthful foods like fruits and vegetables. For those who have a goal of dropping pounds, the TLC diet is a good way to go. In this chapter, we give you the tools you need to make this happen. This includes tips and tricks for not only taking off the weight, but also keeping it off, long term. Here I've supplied you with seven days of 1,200- to

2,000-calorie meal plans. Use these low-calorie menus as a guide to develop your own basic weight-loss diet and then later for weight maintenance.

Losing weight is hard, but keeping the weight off is even harder. It requires vigilance, patience, and commitment, plus the right diet—one that is flexible enough to adapt to any lifestyle and satisfying enough that you won't stray. That's where the TLC diet comes in. It's exactly what you need to be successful and healthy.

Calories in, Calories Out

One pound of fat has 3,500 calories. The standard rule among nutritionists is to reduce your caloric expenditure by 500 calories. This can be via less food, more exercise, or a combination of both. The result is a 1- to 2-pound weight loss a week. Everyone loses weight differently, and we don't usually lose 3,500 calories of pure fat. Generally, if we lose 3,500 calories, some of that is water and some of that is protein. While the majority may be fat, it is never 100 percent. Thus, the 1- to 2-pound cushion does vary, but not by much.

What else should you know about losing weight?

All Calories Are Created Equal (But We Are Not)

A calorie is a calorie is a calorie. This means whether you eat too much fat, too much sugar, too much protein, or even too much broccoli, you will gain weight. No matter where they come from, excess calories will cause you to gain weight. Although it's easier for your body to convert fat to fat, it will still convert protein and carbohydrates (even good carbohydrates) to fat if it doesn't need them.

The reason we focus on fat and sugar when losing weight is that they're the most concentrated source of calories in our diet and the easiest to change. But the truth is, on a weight-loss diet, you should eat less in general, no matter what type of food it is.

Differences in how we manage our weight and our metabolic rate are in our own genetic makeup. This is what allows some people to eat huge amounts of food without gaining a pound, while others seem to just look at food and put on weight (at least, they feel like they do). The same holds true with exercise. In some studies, physical activity caused people to eat more; in others, it made people eat less.

People also vary in how they respond to external food cues, like time or other food triggers, such as eating when bored or tired.

Finally, your body is also very good at adapting to its environment, conserving energy when calorie levels drop and going into starvation mode. Thus, you may be losing weight and then suddenly stop or plateau. This is a sign that you've got to change something if you want to keep losing weight. Changing something means altering or upping your physical activity or adjusting your diet (sometimes people unknowingly return to bad habits and up their caloric intake without realizing it), or both. In any case, something's got to give.

Knowing what kind of person you are and how your body responds to exercise and diet is part of the process of losing and maintaining weight loss. It's something only you can figure out.

How Does This Affect Heart Disease?

While calories are all the same when it comes to weight management, no matter where they come from, that's not the case when it comes to heart disease. Emerging research in the field of nutrition has just begun to look at the effects of specific nutrients on heart disease risk factors. One of the most intriguing and controversial areas surrounds sugar—specifically, fructose in the form of high-fructose corn syrup.

Recent research points to the fact that diets high in high-fructose corn syrup, like that found in drinks, increases both cholesterol and triglyceride levels and raises the risk of heart disease more than other nutrients. Other data shows that people who tend to eat a lot of sugary foods and drinks have more weight around their middle and are more likely to be obese or overweight.

HEALTHFUL LIVING

A small clinical study at the University of California in 2011 compared the effects of consuming 25 percent of their total caloric intake from a sugary drink containing either fructose or high-fructose corn syrup and consuming those same calories from glucose (in the form of bread and crackers). Within two weeks, participants on the sugary drink diet (both fructose and high-fructose corn syrup) had higher levels of LDL cholesterol and triglycerides, putting them at risk for heart disease.

Get Nutrient-Dense

Nutrient-dense foods are foods that are high in nutrients and low in calories. On the TLC diet, you'll be eating a lot of nutrient-dense foods. These are also the kinds of foods that are good for helping you lose weight. Why? They're high in fiber and vitamins and minerals, but not calories. They also fill you up so you're not hungry.

Vegetables top the list of nutrient-dense foods, followed by fruits, beans and dried peas, whole grains, and lean protein. Nutrient-dense foods are the way nature intended. They tend to be whole natural foods, minimally processed.

Don't get confused between energy-dense foods and nutrient-dense foods. *Energy-dense foods* are higher-calorie foods with fewer nutrients. Obvious energy-dense foods are foods like donuts, cookies, cake, and pastries, but also in this category are fruit with heavy syrup, pasta, white bread, and veggies loaded with cheese or cream sauce.

DEFINITION

Nutrient-dense foods are foods that have more beneficial nutrients in relation to calories. In **energy-dense foods,** the foods are high in calories but contain few nutrients, like vitamins, minerals, and fiber.

Given the choice, always choose nutrient-dense over energy-dense foods. For example, apple juice is an energy-dense food supplying lots of calories for little nutrition, compared to an apple, which is a nutrient-dense food. The apple provides 40 percent fewer calories, more than 10 times the amount of fiber, and nearly half the sugar, not to mention other plant compounds we don't even know about.

Developing a Basic Plan

Anytime you start a weight-loss program, either on your own or as a more structured program, you need to have a specific plan in mind. This can be as simple as making one change a week or it can be more elaborate, with planned support meetings and exercise classes. Having a basic plan helps you set and meet goals. It also gets you back on track if you stray.

Set Goals

Setting goals is an important part of any weight-management program. You want your goals to be as specific as possible and short term. Think in terms of two types of goals, process goals and outcome goals. A process goal involves changing a habit or behavior. Examples of some process goals include these:

- Eat more fruits and vegetables.
- Up your intake of whole grains.
- Exercise regularly.

Outcome goals are more specific and focus on a result:

- Lose 10 pounds by the end of the month.
- Run 2 miles three times a week.

Many people focus just on the outcome goals, but you need process goals to achieve and maintain your outcomes. In other words, you need to change behavior and habits to attain your outcome goal. Both are important.

If you're still unsure about how to set and then achieve your goals, try taking the SMART approach: *Specific*, *Measurable*, *Appropriate*, *Realistic*, and *Time-bound.* Every goal should be able to meet SMART standards. Consequently, every goal should be measurable, attainable, and specific. A SMART approach sets you up for success.

Be Realistic

Despite what TV shows like *The Biggest Loser* would have you believe, or what ads touting the newest fad diet or supplement say, no one is going to safely lose 10 or 20 pounds of fat in one week. And no one is going to lose weight while sleeping, working, or not doing anything. In reality, weight loss is a long, slow process that takes hard work and generally months to achieve. Don't be fooled by ads that promise fast weight loss without any work. Remember, slow and steady wins the race!

Be realistic about how much you want to lose and what it will take to lose it. Most people will never look like the skinny celebrities or models on television, no matter how hard they try—nor should they strive to be like them.

When it comes to heart health, all it takes is a small weight loss (10 to 15 pounds) even in an obese person to see major improvements in blood lipid levels (as well as blood sugar levels and blood pressure). Your main focus is on *your health* and how you feel, not what you look like. Always keep that goal in mind. Stay focused, and you will be successful and able to weather any stresses (financial, relationship, and so on).

In a perfect world, you would never gain back a pound or go off your diet, but that's not going to happen. Expect to slip up now and then—and maybe even gain back a few pounds. This is normal. The key to success is not letting any of these setbacks get out of control. Go back to the TLC diet, even if you were off for a few days, and don't let a few pounds derail you from your goal. Remember how good you feel, focus on the benefits of your good health, and keep on trying.

Don't Skip Meals

Some people feel that the easiest way to cut calories is simply to skip a meal. This way, they will not be tempted to eat more and they won't have to worry about portions. *Wrong!* Skipping meals is one of the worst things you can do, both mentally and physically.

When you skip a meal, you may feel like you can eat more at your next meal, to make up for the lost calories earlier. In some people, this "rebound" effect ends in overeating at the next meal, as you feel the need to "compensate" for these calories. Physically, skipping meals—particularly if you're skipping breakfast or if it's been a long period of time since your last meal—forces the body into a "fasting" state. In this state, your metabolism slows and energy is conserved, meaning that when you do eat again, any excess is more likely to be stored as fat (as your body is preparing for another fasting state).

Finally, if you are skipping a meal that you normally eat simply to lose weight, don't bother. Not only will this sabotage you both physically and psychologically, but this is a practice that just won't work in the long term. Eat your normal meal or a small meal instead.

Keep Track of Your Weight

Keeping track of your weight during the weight loss process is crucial for success, but it's just as important after the fact, for weight maintenance. As I mentioned earlier, you may gain back a few pounds, but that's okay as long as your health and your blood lipids, blood sugar, and blood pressure continue to be in good shape. The key is to not keep regaining until the benefits of losing weight are gone.

The calorie level that's right for maintaining your weight largely depends on your own individual body. In studies on weight loss from Columbia University, we know that people who lose large amounts of weight (about 10 percent of their total body weight or more) are metabolically different from those people who have never lost weight. As a result, they need to eat less and exercise more than their never-lost-weight counterparts, some 20 percent less than normal. This means someone who would typically need 1,500 calories to maintain their normal weight would require only 1,200 calories to maintain this same amount of weight if that person had lost a lot of weight. To increase caloric levels, you need to increase physical activity to compensate. Adding that extra 20 percent would cause the weight to creep back up over a year or so.

Aside from eating less and exercising more, successful losers have some other common characteristics, as noted by the National Weight Control Registry (NWCR). The NWCR tracks more than 10,000 people who have lost significant amounts of weight and kept it off for long periods of time. To be eligible to join, you need to have lost at least 30 pounds and kept it off for one year or longer. See the website at nwcr.ws for more information.

HEALTHFUL LIVING

The average member in the National Weight Control Registry has lost more than 70 pounds and remained at that weight for five years or more.

Here's what they have in common:

- Exercise regularly, about an hour or more a day
- Eat a diet low in fat and calories (around 50 to 300 fewer calories than people their same size)
- Eat breakfast regularly
- Weigh themselves every day
- Don't cheat (catch slips before they snowball)
- Eat a consistent diet

The best advice for your heart and your health is to prevent the pounds from piling on in the first place, but if that's not the case, all is not lost. While losing weight may be a long and tedious process, it is still well worth the effort and reward of a long, healthy, high-quality life, particularly in your older years.

Seven-Day Weight Loss Menu Plan

Here are the seven-day diets for 1,200, 1,500, 1,800, and 2,000 calories. All the menus are under 7 percent calories from saturated fat and 200 milligrams of cholesterol, and fall into the range of 25 to 35 percent total fat or less and under 2,300 milligrams of sodium.

Fiber levels are high, as high-fiber diets and particularly soluble fiber (see Chapter 14) are beneficial for people trying to lower their cholesterol. If you experience gastrointestinal problems, reduce the fiber by lowering your intake of high-fiber foods like beans, nuts, and whole grains and replacing them with more refined products similar in calories like fruit juice, white pasta, rice, and crackers. Then gradually try to reintroduce those high-fiber foods into your diet. The goal is to increase your soluble fiber so you can regularly include high-fiber foods like whole grains (oatmeal is a good example), beans, and nuts in your diet. At the same time you need to be at a level you feel comfortable with and can tolerate.

Increasing the Calories of Each Diet

The backbone of the plan is the 1,200-calorie diet. It is used as the basis for the 1,500-, 1,800-, and 2,000-calorie diets. Calories are increased in 200 or 300 increments by increasing portion sizes (for example, from three carrot sticks to six carrot sticks) or adding a few more foods. I've put these higher-calorie foods in *italics* to let you know what in the diet has changed. This way you can adapt your meal plan to any calorie level with just a few simple changes.

Flexibility

These meal plans are meant to help you understand the pattern or style of eating the TLC way. You may not like all the foods, and that's okay—these menus have flexibility built in. You can substitute a food or ingredient as long as it is in the same food group and is similar in calories. This keeps you following the pattern. There may be slight differences in calories, but most of the time, these are negligible. For instance, if you don't like beef, you can use lean pork instead, or if you don't eat red meat, substitute chicken. Here are some other foods for which you have flexibility.

Fruits and vegetables. These can vary from season to season. Thus, in the fall and winter, you may be leaning toward cauliflower, broccoli, and brussels sprouts; in the summer, it's tomatoes, peppers, and zucchini. Fruit, although now available all year long (particularly if you buy it frozen), is still best during its peak season. You can pretty much substitute any vegetable or fruit for another. The exception is avocado, which is high in fat.

Vegetable oils. In this book, I use corn oil, canola oil, and olive oil, but you can use almost any polyunsaturated or monounsaturated oil you like. If I do specify olive oil, it's more for the flavor than the fat.

Nuts. With the exception of only a few high-fat nuts, like macadamia nuts and Brazil nuts, most tree nuts can easily be interchanged. They do vary in size, which affects amount.

Milk. Most milk is listed as nonfat or skim cow's milk, but you can choose low-fat (1 percent) cow's milk, unsweetened soy milk, or unsweetened low-fat almond milk. Although slightly different in nutrient content, they do not vary by huge amounts.

Eggs. All these menus use egg whites in place of whole eggs, but if you've gotten your cholesterol down, have healthy blood lipid levels, and are following the TLC diet, it's okay to have a whole egg once in a while. In some of the recipes, you may see four egg whites for two servings. Here, you may want to use one whole egg and two egg whites in place of the four egg whites.

Creativity

Use these menus as a guide to introduce you to different foods and a world of herbs and spices. Don't be afraid to explore new ingredients and experiment with different flavor combinations or cooking methods. Let your imagination go as your cooking skills grow. For example, take the traditional hummus. You can opt for a flavored variety, like garlic or red pepper, or you can make your own, with black beans or edamame replacing the chickpeas. The sky's the limit when it comes to creating new dishes.

Leftovers Management

In this seven-day menu, notice that meals often appear more than once—and sometimes even three times during the week. There are several reasons for this. First and foremost is that it cuts down on work in the kitchen. It also makes life easier. Cook once, eat twice (or more) saves time and money. Soup is a great example of a meal that is ideal for this kind of menu management. These foods are so good you won't mind having them again!

The Recipes

The recipes you'll see in initial caps (such as Overnight Pineapple Coconut Oatmeal) are included in Part 4. You'll also find many more recipes there for tasty breakfasts, snacks, fast and easy entrées, vegetarian dishes, desserts, and more.

Day 1

1,200 Calories

1,221 calories, 41 g fat, 7 g saturated fat, 28 mg cholesterol, 33 g fiber, 807 mg sodium

56 percent carbs, 28 percent fat, 16 percent protein

Breakfast: Overnight Pineapple Coconut Oatmeal

Snack: 3 carrot sticks, 6 celery sticks, 2 TB. hummus

Lunch: 4 cups chopped green leaf lettuce; 1/2 medium tomato, cut in wedges; 1/2 cucumber, sliced; 1/2 cup sliced mushrooms; 1/2 cup cooked chickpeas; dressing: 1 tsp. olive oil and 2 tsp. balsamic vinegar, salt and pepper to taste

Snack: 1 medium apple; 2 TB. all-natural, unsalted peanut butter

Dinner: 1 serving Maple-Glazed Scallops with Sautéed Spinach, 3/4 cup cooked wild rice blend

1,500 Calories

1,523 calories, 49 g fat, 8 g saturated fat, 28 mg cholesterol, 36 g fiber, 1,091 mg sodium

59 percent carbs, 27 percent fat, 14 percent protein

Breakfast: Overnight Pineapple Coconut Oatmeal

Snack: 3 carrot sticks, 6 celery sticks, 2 TB. hummus

Lunch: 4 cups chopped green leaf lettuce; 1/2 medium tomato, cut in wedges; 1/2 cucumber, sliced; 1/2 cup sliced mushrooms; 1/2 cup cooked chickpeas; dressing: 1 tsp. olive oil and 2 tsp. balsamic vinegar, salt and pepper to taste; *1 medium apple; 2 TB. all-natural, unsalted peanut butter*

Snack: *1 Morning Glory Muffin, 1 TB. jelly, 2 rice cakes*

Dinner: 1 serving Maple-Glazed Scallops with Sautéed Spinach, 3/4 cup cooked wild rice blend

1,800 Calories

1,789 calories, 56 g fat, 11 g saturated fat, 88 mg cholesterol, 38 g fiber, 1,375 mg sodium

55 percent carbs, 27 percent fat, 18 percent protein

Breakfast: Overnight Pineapple Coconut Oatmeal; *1 cup 1 percent milk; 1 cup coffee with remaining milk, 1 packet sugar*

Snack: *6* carrot sticks, 6 celery sticks, *1/4 cup* hummus

Lunch: 4 cups chopped green leaf lettuce; 1/2 medium tomato, cut in wedges; 1/2 cucumber, sliced; 1/2 cup sliced mushrooms; 1/2 cup cooked chickpeas; *2 oz. cooked chicken breast, chopped;* dressing: 1 tsp. olive oil and 2 tsp. balsamic vinegar, salt and pepper to taste; *1 medium apple; 2 TB. all-natural, unsalted peanut butter*

Snack: *1 Morning Glory Muffin, 1 TB. jelly, 2 rice cakes*

Dinner: 1 serving Maple-Glazed Scallops with Sautéed Spinach, 3/4 cup cooked wild rice blend

2,000 Calories

1,993 calories, 63 g fat, 12 g saturated fat, 112 mg cholesterol, 39 g fiber, 1,399 mg sodium

53 percent carbs, 27 percent fat, 20 percent protein

Breakfast: Overnight Pineapple Coconut Oatmeal; *1 cup 1 percent milk; 1 cup coffee with remaining milk, 1 packet sugar*

Snack: *6* carrot sticks, 6 celery sticks, *1/4 cup* hummus

Lunch: 4 cups chopped green leaf lettuce; 1/2 medium tomato, cut in wedges; 1/2 cucumber, sliced; 1/2 cup sliced mushrooms; 1/2 cup cooked chickpeas; *3 oz. cooked chicken breast, chopped;* dressing: 1 tsp. olive oil and 2 tsp. balsamic vinegar, salt and pepper to taste; *1 medium apple; 2 TB all-natural, unsalted peanut butter*

Snack: *1 Morning Glory Muffin, 1 TB. jelly, 2 rice cakes*

Dinner: 1 serving Maple-Glazed Scallops with Sautéed Spinach, $^3/_4$ cup cooked wild rice blend, *$^1/_2$ cup TLC Chocolate Pudding with 2 medium whole strawberries and 5 whole almonds, crushed*

Day 2

1,200 Calories

1,212 calories, 32 g fat, 5 g saturated fat, 47 mg cholesterol, 34 g fiber, 1,162 mg sodium

54 percent carbs, 23 percent fat, 23 percent protein

Breakfast: $^1/_4$ cup each chopped onion, red pepper, and green pepper, sautéed in 1 tsp. olive oil and scrambled with 3 egg whites; 1 whole-wheat English muffin with 2 tsp. soft margarine fortified with sterols

Snack: Black and Blue Vanilla Smoothie

Lunch: 1 serving Curried Chicken Salad, whole-wheat roll

Snack: $^1/_2$ cup nonfat Greek-style yogurt, 1 TB. peanut butter or almond butter, 1 banana

Dinner: 3 oz. broiled salmon topped with 1 medium orange, sectioned, mixed with 2 TB. chopped cilantro and 5 whole almonds, crushed, and $^1/_2$ tsp olive oil; 1 medium baked sweet potato; 6 steamed broccoli spears

1,500 Calories

1,496 calories, 43 g fat, 8 g saturated fat, 66 mg cholesterol, 37 g fiber, 1,397 mg sodium

52 percent carbs, 25 percent fat, 23 percent protein

Breakfast: $^1/_4$ cup each chopped onion, red pepper, and green pepper, 1 cup raw sliced mushrooms sautéed in 1 tsp. olive oil and scrambled with 3 egg whites; 1 whole-wheat English muffin with 2 tsp. soft margarine fortified with sterols; *6 oz. orange juice*

Snack: Black and Blue Vanilla Smoothie

Lunch: 1 serving Curried Chicken Salad, whole-wheat roll

Snack: $\frac{1}{2}$ cup nonfat Greek-style yogurt, 1 TB. peanut butter or almond butter, 1 banana

Dinner: 3 oz. broiled salmon topped with 1 medium orange, sectioned, mixed with 2 TB. chopped cilantro and 5 whole almonds, crushed, and $\frac{1}{2}$ tsp olive oil; 1 medium baked sweet potato; 6 steamed broccoli spears; *1 serving Watermelon Feta Salad*

1,800 Calories

1,807 calories, 55 g fat, 12 g saturated fat, 102 mg cholesterol, 39 g fiber, 1,205 mg sodium

52 percent carbs, 26 percent fat, 22 percent protein

Breakfast: $\frac{1}{4}$ cup each chopped onion, red pepper, and green pepper, 1 cup raw sliced mushrooms sautéed in 1 tsp. olive oil and scrambled with 3 egg whites; 1 whole-wheat English muffin with 2 tsp. soft margarine fortified with sterols; *8 oz. orange juice*

Snack: Black and Blue Vanilla Smoothie

Lunch: 1 serving Curried Chicken Salad, whole-wheat roll, *1 cup diced steamed summer squash, 2 cups diced honeydew melon*

Snack: *1 cup* low-fat Greek-style yogurt, *2 TB.* peanut butter or almond butter, 1 banana

Dinner: 3 oz. broiled salmon topped with 1 medium orange, sectioned, mixed with 2 TB. chopped cilantro, 5 whole almonds, crushed, and $\frac{1}{2}$ tsp olive oil; 1 large baked sweet potato; *$1\frac{1}{2}$ cups steamed broccoli and cauliflower florets; 3 cups air-popped popcorn sprinkled with chili powder or cinnamon; 1 serving Watermelon Feta Salad*

2,000 Calories

1,993 calories, 62 g fat, 13 g saturated fat, 103 mg cholesterol, 39 g fiber, 1,517 mg sodium

52 percent carbs, 27 percent fat, 21 percent protein

Breakfast: $\frac{1}{4}$ cup each chopped onion, red pepper, and green pepper, 1 cup raw sliced mushrooms sautéed in 1 tsp. olive oil and scrambled with 3 egg whites; 1 whole-wheat English muffin with 2 tsp. soft margarine fortified with sterols; *8 oz. orange juice*

Snack: Black and Blue Vanilla Smoothie, *5 saltine crackers*

Lunch: 1 serving Curried Chicken Salad, *plain white dinner roll, 1 cup diced steamed summer squash, 2 cups diced honeydew melon*

Snack: *1 cup* low-fat Greek-style yogurt, *2 TB.* peanut butter or almond butter, 1 banana

Dinner: 3 oz. broiled salmon topped with 1 *small* orange, sectioned, mixed with 2 TB. chopped cilantro, 5 whole almonds, crushed, and $^1/_2$ tsp. olive oil; *1 medium baked, peeled, and mashed sweet potato; $1^1/_2$ cups steamed broccoli and cauliflower florets; 3 cups air-popped popcorn sprinkled with chili powder or cinnamon with 1 tsp. melted soft margarine fortified with plant sterols; 1 serving Watermelon Feta Salad*

Day 3

1,200 Calories

1,212 calories, 26 g fat, 6 g saturated fat, 79 mg cholesterol, 26 g fiber, 1,622 mg sodium

57 percent carbs, 19 percent fat, 24 percent protein

Breakfast: Overnight Pineapple Coconut Oatmeal

Snack: 1 cup Tomato Basil White Bean Soup

Lunch: 2 oz. low-sodium deli turkey breast; 1 slice ($^3/_4$ oz.) sliced low-fat processed Swiss cheese on kaiser roll with 1 slice tomato, 1 piece lettuce, and 1 TB. canola mayonnaise

Snack: $^1/_4$ mango, sliced; 6 oz. 1 percent milk

Dinner: 1 serving Tilapia with Summer Squash, $^3/_4$ cup whole-wheat cooked spaghetti

1,500 Calories

1,497 calories, 36 g fat, 8 g saturated fat, 89 mg cholesterol, 36 g fiber, 1,959 mg sodium

56 percent carbs, 21 percent fat, 23 percent protein

Breakfast: Overnight Pineapple Coconut Oatmeal

Snack: 1 cup Tomato Basil White Bean Soup *topped with 3 oz. chopped avocado*

Lunch: 2 oz. low-sodium deli turkey breast; *2 slices* (3/4 oz. each) low-fat processed Swiss cheese on kaiser roll with *2 slices* tomato, *2 pieces* lettuce, and 1 TB. canola mayonnaise

Snack: 1/2 mango, sliced; *1 cup* 1 percent milk

Dinner: 1 serving Tilapia with Summer Squash, *1 cup* whole-wheat cooked spaghetti

1,800 Calories

1,825 calories, 44 g fat, 9 g saturated fat, 107 mg cholesterol, 38 g fiber, 2,199 mg sodium

58 percent carbs, 21 percent fat, 21 percent protein

Breakfast: Overnight Pineapple Coconut Oatmeal

Snack: 1 cup Tomato Basil White Bean Soup *topped with 3 oz. chopped avocado*

Lunch: 2 oz. low-sodium deli turkey breast; *2 slices* low-fat processed Swiss cheese on kaiser roll with *2 slices* tomato, *2 pieces* lettuce, and 1 TB. canola mayonnaise

Snack: 1/2 mango, sliced; *1 cup* 1 percent milk

Dinner: 1 serving Tilapia with Summer Squash, *1 1/2 cups spaghetti, 1 cup sliced strawberries, 1 piece Pumpkin Ginger Bread*

2,000 Calories

1,983 calories, 52 g fat, 10 g saturated fat, 92 mg cholesterol, 38 g fiber, 1,619 mg sodium

59 percent carbs, 22 percent fat, 19 percent protein

Breakfast: Overnight Pineapple Coconut Oatmeal

Snack: 1 cup Tomato Basil White Bean Soup *topped with 3 oz. chopped avocado*

Lunch: 2 oz. low-sodium deli turkey breast; *2 slices* low-fat processed Swiss cheese on kaiser roll with *2 slices* tomato, *2 pieces* lettuce, and *2 tsp. mustard*

Snack: 1/2 mango, sliced; *1 oz. (about 18) cashews; 1 cup* 1 percent milk

Dinner: 1 serving Tilapia with Summer Squash, *2 cups spaghetti, 3/4 cup diced cantaloupe, 1 piece Pumpkin Ginger Bread*

Day 4

1,200 Calories

1,203 calories, 35 g fat, 6 g saturated fat, 12 mg cholesterol, 31 g fiber, 863 mg sodium

59 percent carbs, 25 percent fat, 16 percent protein

Breakfast: ³⁄₄ cup bran cereal, 1 cup 1 percent milk

Snack: 4 low-fat cinnamon graham crackers with 1 TB. almond butter

Lunch: 1 serving Asparagus with Sun-Dried Tomatoes, Quinoa, and Basmati Rice; ¹⁄₂ cup cooked red beans; 1 plum

Snack: Black and Blue Vanilla Smoothie with 1 TB. ground flaxseeds, 10 grapes

Dinner: 1 cup Spicy Tofu and Green Bean Stir-Fry, ³⁄₄ cup brown rice sprinkled with 1 TB. sunflower seeds

1,500 Calories

1,496 calories, 50 g fat, 8 g saturated fat, 12 mg cholesterol, 37 g fiber, 1,091 mg sodium

56 percent carbs, 29 percent fat, 15 percent protein

Breakfast: ³⁄₄ cup bran cereal, 1 cup 1 percent milk, *1 apple, peeled and diced*

Snack: 4 low-fat cinnamon graham crackers with *2 TB.* almond butter

Lunch: 1 serving Asparagus with Sun-Dried Tomatoes, Quinoa, and Basmati Rice; ¹⁄₂ cup cooked red beans; 1 plum

Snack: Black and Blue Vanilla Smoothie with 1 TB. ground flaxseeds, 10 grapes

Dinner: *2 cups* Spicy Tofu and Green Bean Stir-Fry, ³⁄₄ cup brown rice sprinkled with 1 TB. sunflower seeds

1,800 Calories

1,814 calories, 63 g fat, 10 g saturated fat, 14 mg cholesterol, 40 g fiber, 1,864 mg sodium

53 percent carbs, 30 percent fat, 17 percent protein

Breakfast: $^3/_4$ cup bran cereal, 1 cup 1 percent milk, *1 apple, peeled and diced*

Snack: 4 low-fat cinnamon graham crackers with *2 TB.* almond butter

Lunch: 1 serving Asparagus with Sun-Dried Tomatoes, Quinoa, and Basmati Rice; $^1/_2$ cup cooked red beans; *1 grilled veggie burger on hamburger bun with 1 TB. ketchup and 1 TB. low-fat canola mayonnaise;* 1 plum

Snack: Black and Blue Vanilla Smoothie with 1 TB. ground flaxseeds, 10 grapes

Dinner: *2 cups* Spicy Tofu and Green Bean Stir-Fry, $^3/_4$ cup brown rice sprinkled with 1 TB. sunflower seeds

2,000 Calories

1,996 calories, 70 g fat, 13 g saturated fat, 32 mg cholesterol, 41 g fiber, 2,159 mg sodium

53 percent carbs, 30 percent fat, 17 percent protein

Breakfast: $^3/_4$ cup bran cereal, 1 cup 1 percent milk, *1 apple, peeled and diced*

Snack: *8* low-fat cinnamon graham crackers with *2 TB.* almond butter

Lunch: 1 serving Asparagus with Sun-Dried Tomatoes, Quinoa, and Basmati Rice; $^1/_2$ cup cooked red beans; *1 grilled veggie burger on hamburger bun with 1 TB. ketchup, 1 TB. low-fat canola mayonnaise, 2 slices tomato, 2 pieces lettuce, and 1 oz. sliced avocado;* 1 plum

Snack: Black and Blue Vanilla Smoothie, 10 grapes, *1 oz. low-fat mozzarella string cheese*

Dinner: *2 cups* Spicy Tofu and Green Bean Stir-Fry, *1 cup rice noodles* sprinkled with 1 TB. sunflower seeds

Day 5

1,200 Calories

1,211 calories, 27 g fat, 4 g saturated fat, 80 mg cholesterol, 34 g fiber, 695 mg sodium

59 percent carbs, 20 percent fat, 21 percent protein

Breakfast: Banana Oatmeal Peanut Butter Shake

Snack: 1 piece Pumpkin Ginger Bread, 1 orange

Lunch: 1 serving Tilapia with Summer Squash, $^3/_4$ cup cooked quinoa

Snack: 1 cup cooked chickpeas with $^1/_2$ oz. low-fat feta cheese, 1 tsp. olive oil, and 1 tsp. lemon juice

Dinner: 1 serving Curried Chicken Salad

1,500 Calories

1,485 calories, 40 g fat, 8 g saturated fat, 98 mg cholesterol, 38 g fiber, 781 mg sodium

54 percent carbs, 24 percent fat, 22 percent protein

Breakfast: Banana Oatmeal Peanut Butter Shake, *1 serving Cranberry Nut Muesli*

Snack: 1 piece Pumpkin Ginger Bread, 1 orange

Lunch: 1 serving Tilapia with Summer Squash, $^3/_4$ cup cooked quinoa, *$^1/_2$ cup 1 percent low-fat yogurt with 1 tsp. honey*

Snack: 1 cup cooked chickpeas with *$^1/_4$ cup chopped red pepper,* $^1/_2$ oz. low-fat feta cheese, 1 tsp. olive oil, and 1 tsp. lemon juice

Dinner: 1 serving Curried Chicken Salad

1,800 Calories

1,794 calories, 44 g fat, 9 g saturated fat, 118 mg cholesterol, 40 g fiber, 1,397 mg sodium

56 percent carbs, 22 percent fat, 22 percent protein

Breakfast: Banana Oatmeal Peanut Butter Shake, *1 serving Cranberry Nut Muesli*

Snack: 1 piece Pumpkin Ginger Bread, 1 small orange

Lunch: 1 serving Tilapia with Summer Squash, $^3/_4$ cup cooked quinoa, *$^1/_2$ cup 1 percent low-fat yogurt with 1 tsp. honey*

Snack: 1 cup cooked chickpeas with *$^1/_4$ cup chopped red pepper, 1 oz.* low-fat feta cheese, 1 tsp. olive oil, and 1 tsp. lemon juice

Dinner: *2 servings* Curried Chicken Salad, *1 large pita, $1^1/_2$ cups diced watermelon*

2,000 Calories

2,003 calories, 53 g fat, 11 g saturated fat, 123 mg cholesterol, 41 g fiber, 1,472 mg sodium

55 percent carbs, 23 percent fat, 22 percent protein

Breakfast: Banana Oatmeal Peanut Butter Shake, *1 serving Cranberry Nut Muesli*

Snack: 1 piece Pumpkin Ginger Bread, 1 small orange

Lunch: 1 serving Tilapia with Summer Squash, ¾ cup cooked quinoa, *½ cup 1 percent low-fat yogurt with 1 tsp. honey*

Snack: 1 cup cooked chickpeas with *¼ cup chopped red pepper, 1 oz.* low-fat feta cheese, *2 tsp.* olive oil, and 1 tsp. lemon juice

Dinner: *2 servings* Curried Chicken Salad, *1 large pita, 1½ cups diced watermelon, 1 No-Bake Peanut Butter Oatmeal Cookie*

Day 6

1,200 Calories

1,206 calories, 34 g fat, 6 g saturated fat, 89 mg cholesterol, 22 g fiber, 1,475 mg sodium

51 percent carbs, 24 percent fat, 25 percent protein

Breakfast: Spinach-Egg-Potato Scramble, 8 oz. orange juice

Snack: 1 apple, 1 TB. almond butter

Lunch: Grilled Eggplant and Tomato Panini

Snack: 1 cup cantaloupe with ½ cup low-fat cottage cheese

Dinner: 3 oz. diced chicken breast sautéed with 1 tsp. corn oil, 3 cups raw baby spinach, and 1 cup raw sliced mushrooms; 1 small boiled potato, diced, sprinkled with 1 TB. Parmesan cheese

1,500 Calories

1,508 calories, 45 g fat, 9 g saturated fat, 95 mg cholesterol, 29 g fiber, 1,554 mg sodium

51 percent carbs, 26 percent fat, 23 percent protein

Breakfast: Spinach-Egg-Potato Scramble, 8 oz. orange juice

Snack: 1 apple, 1 TB. almond butter, *1 serving Cranberry Nut Muesli with $^1/_2$ cup 1 percent milk, 1 cup blueberries*

Lunch: Grilled Eggplant and Tomato Panini

Snack: 1 cup cantaloupe with $^1/_2$ cup low-fat cottage cheese

Dinner: 3 oz. diced chicken breast sautéed with 1 tsp. corn oil, 3 cups raw baby spinach, and 1 cup raw sliced mushrooms; 1 small boiled potato, diced, sprinkled with 1 TB. Parmesan cheese

1,800 Calories

1,800 calories, 53 g fat, 10 g saturated fat, 100 mg cholesterol, 34 g fiber, 2,078 mg sodium

51 percent carbs, 25 percent fat, 24 percent protein

Breakfast: Spinach-Egg-Potato Scramble, 8 oz. orange juice

Snack: 1 apple, 1 TB. almond butter, *1 serving Cranberry Nut Muesli with $^1/_2$ cup 1 percent milk, 1 cup blueberries*

Lunch: Grilled Eggplant and Tomato Panini

Snack: *2 cups pineapple with 1 cup* low-fat cottage cheese

Dinner: 3 oz. diced chicken breast sautéed with 1 tsp. corn oil, *3 cups raw chopped kale*, and 1 cup sliced raw mushrooms; 1 small boiled potato, diced, sprinkled with 1 TB. Parmesan cheese; *2 cups chopped lettuce, $^1/_2$ cucumber, sliced; $^1/_2$ small red onion; dressing: 1 tsp. olive oil and 1 tsp. balsamic vinegar*

2,000 Calories

1,994 calories, 59 g fat, 11 g saturated fat, 106 mg cholesterol, 39 g fiber, 2,140 mg sodium

53 percent carbs, 25 percent fat, 24 percent protein

Breakfast: Spinach-Egg-Potato Scramble, 8 oz. orange juice

Snack: 1 apple, 1 TB. almond butter, *1 serving Cranberry Nut Muesli with ½ cup 1 percent milk, 1 cup blueberries*

Lunch: Grilled Eggplant and Tomato Panini

Snack: *2 cups pineapple with 1 cup* low-fat cottage cheese *and 5 pecan halves*

Dinner: 3 oz. diced chicken breast sautéed with 1 tsp. corn oil, *3 cups raw chopped kale,* and 1 cup sliced raw mushrooms; *½ cup cooked diced carrots;* 1 small boiled potato, diced, sprinkled with 1 TB. Parmesan cheese; *3 cups chopped lettuce, ½ cucumber, sliced; ½ small red onion; dressing: 1 tsp. olive oil and 1 tsp. balsamic vinegar*

Day 7

1,200 Calories

1,196 calories, 33 g fat, 7 g saturated fat, 78 mg cholesterol, 35 g fiber, 1,552 mg sodium

54 percent carbs, 23 percent fat, 23 percent protein

Breakfast: Fruit salad: ½ cup each raspberries, blueberries, strawberries, and blackberries, mixed with ½ cup 1 percent low-fat yogurt and ⅓ cup bran flakes

Snack: 4 TB. hummus, 15 whole-wheat crackers

Lunch: 1 cup Spicy Tofu and Green Bean Stir-Fry, 1 cup Japanese soba noodles, ½ mango, sliced

Snack: 1 piece Pumpkin Ginger Bread

Dinner: 3 oz. sirloin steak, cut into strips and stir-fried with 1 tsp. sesame seed oil, 1 clove crushed garlic, 1 cup cooked chopped broccoli, 1 cup sliced red or green pepper, and ½ cup sliced onion, tossed with 1 tsp. low-sodium soy sauce, 1 tsp. water, and 1 tsp. hot sauce

1,500 Calories

1,516 calories, 39 g fat, 7 g saturated fat, 78 mg cholesterol, 39 g fiber, 1,620 mg sodium

57 percent carbs, 22 percent fat, 21 percent protein

Breakfast: Fruit salad: $1/2$ cup each raspberries, blueberries, strawberries, and blackberries, mixed with $1/2$ cup 1 percent low-fat yogurt, $1/3$ cup bran flakes, and *10 whole almonds, crushed*

Snack: 4 TB. hummus, 15 whole-wheat crackers

Lunch: 1 cup Spicy Tofu and Green Bean Stir-Fry, *2 cups* Japanese soba noodles, $1/2$ mango, sliced

Snack: 1 piece Pumpkin Ginger Bread

Dinner: 3 oz. sirloin steak, cut into strips and stir-fried with 1 tsp. sesame seed oil, 1 clove crushed garlic, 1 cup cooked chopped broccoli, 1 cup sliced red or green pepper, and $1/2$ cup sliced onion, tossed with 1 tsp. low-sodium soy sauce, 1 tsp. water, and 1 tsp. hot sauce; *$3/4$ cup cooked wild rice*

1,800 Calories

1,816 calories, 49 g fat, 9 g saturated fat, 96 mg cholesterol, 39 g fiber, 1,966 mg sodium

55 percent carbs, 23 percent fat, 22 percent protein

Breakfast: Fruit salad: $1/2$ cup each raspberries, blueberries, strawberries, and blackberries, mixed with *1 cup* 1 percent low-fat yogurt, $1/3$ cup bran flakes, and *10 whole almonds, crushed*

Snack: 4 TB. hummus, *8 multigrain flaxseed crackers*

Lunch: 2 cups Spicy Tofu and Green Bean Stir-Fry, *2 cups Japanese soba noodles*, $1/2$ mango, sliced

Snack: 1 piece Pumpkin Ginger Bread, *6 oz. vanilla soy milk*

Dinner: 3 oz. sirloin steak, cut into strips and stir-fried with 1 tsp. sesame seed oil, *1 tsp. corn oil*, 1 clove crushed garlic, 1 cup cooked chopped broccoli, 1 cup sliced red or green pepper, and $1/2$ cup sliced onion, tossed with 1 tsp. low-sodium soy sauce, 1 tsp. water, and 1 tsp. hot sauce; *$3/4$ cup steamed white sticky rice*

2,000 Calories

2,008 calories, 56 g fat, 11 g saturated fat, 90 mg cholesterol, 39.5 g fiber, 1,735 mg sodium

55 percent carbs, 25 percent fat, 22 percent protein

Breakfast: Fruit salad: $\frac{1}{2}$ cup each raspberries, blueberries, strawberries, and blackberries, mixed with *1 cup* 1 percent low-fat yogurt, $\frac{1}{4}$ cup bran flakes, and *10 whole almonds, crushed*

Snack: *$1\frac{1}{2}$ cups Tuna and Apple Salad, 8 multigrain flaxseed crackers*

Lunch: 2 cups Spicy Tofu and Green Bean Stir-Fry, *2 cups Japanese soba noodles,* $\frac{1}{2}$ mango, sliced

Snack: *2 No-Bake Peanut Butter Oatmeal Cookies, 1 cup vanilla soy milk; 1 pink grapefruit cut in half and sprinkled with 2 tsp. brown sugar*

Dinner: 3 oz. sirloin steak, cut into strips and stir-fried with 1 tsp. sesame seed oil, *1 tsp. corn oil,* 1 clove crushed garlic, 1 cup cooked chopped broccoli, 1 cup sliced red or green pepper, and $\frac{1}{2}$ cup sliced onion, tossed with 1 tsp. low-sodium soy sauce, 1 tsp. water, and 1 tsp. hot sauce; *$\frac{3}{4}$ cup steamed white sticky rice*

The Least You Need to Know

- Losing weight and keeping the weight off takes time and vigilance.
- The TLC diet focuses on nutrient-dense foods that are high in nutrients and low in calories, like high-fiber vegetables and whole grains.
- Be sure to set realistic goals and then stick to them.
- Don't skip meals if you're trying to lose weight.
- The TLC diet has a flexible meal pattern that allows you to mix and match foods to meet your individual needs and preferences.

Chapter 11

Savvy Substitutions

In This Chapter

- Making smarter food choices
- Why low-fat and fat-free foods aren't necessarily good
- Cutting the fat, sugar, dairy, and salt in recipes
- Simple swaps to remember

When it comes to eating healthfully, you don't always have to make major overhauls in your diet. Sometimes all it takes is a simple substitution of one ingredient or food for another. At first, this may seem challenging—maybe even burdensome—but as you get used to it, it will become second nature.

Furthermore, as you get into the habit of making one substitution—say, switching from white bread to whole-grain bread—you'll eventually find it easier to do another, like switching from whole milk to low-fat or nonfat milk. Remember, too, you don't have to sub out every single high-fat or high-calorie food you eat—at least, not at first. As you begin to eat more healthfully, however, these higher-fat foods will begin to lose their appeal, and you'll reach for the better option without even thinking about it.

If you think of your TLC diet simply as swapping out high-fat foods for lower-fat foods, or giving up refined carbs in favor of complex carbs, the changes won't seem so overwhelming or so drastic. In fact, swapping out less nutritious food for healthier versions is relatively easy and practically foolproof. In the next few pages, I give you plenty of ideas for how to do this.

Sometimes, however, there are bumps in the road and what looks like a good substitution really isn't. I talk about that, too, and give you some ways to avoid falling into those traps.

Finally, I share some of the tricks of the trade for making ingredient substitutions in baking and making other recipes, like sauces. While these can be tricky, some guidelines make it easier to start. At the end of this chapter is also a handy list you can pull out when you're not sure what substitutions work best.

Finding More Healthful Versions of High-Fat Foods

When it comes to swapping out less nutritious food for better choices, think about going for natural, wholesome foods—foods that are closest to their natural state and foods that are least processed. This is the golden rule of healthful substitutions. Some examples of this: in lieu of french fries, have a baked potato; for macaroni and cheese, opt for whole-grain pasta with tomato sauce and a sprinkle of Parmesan cheese; and in place of a Caesar salad, choose a plain salad that you dress yourself with an oil-and-vinegar dressing. Keep this in mind, and you can't go wrong.

If you focus on cutting the saturated fat, trans fats, and cholesterol in your diet and your foods, you will automatically reduce calories, which can help you lose weight. Focusing on all-natural, unprocessed foods also will cut calories *and* curb your added sugar and salt intake, two other nutrients that can hurt your heart.

To keep from being trapped with poor choices and few healthful options, like at the office, consider bringing your lunch to work on a regular basis. Make it a point to pack a healthful lunch, including fruit, lean meat, and some vegetables, three or four days a week. Not only will this be better for your heart, but it can also save you money in the long run. Consider that bringing in lunch just two days a week would save you about $10 to $15 a week; then multiply that by 50, to get a savings of as much as $750 a year.

GOTCHA!

Many people mistakenly switch from one processed food to another, such as from a regular canned soup to a low-sodium version, or from pepperoni pizza to plain cheese pizza. While this is okay if you don't have any other healthful options, ideally, you want to go from a canned soup to a homemade version or from pepperoni pizza to a less processed meal, like lean chicken breast with mashed sweet potatoes and green beans.

If you do find yourself in a fast-food restaurant or any restaurant with limited options, you can make some healthful choices. Consider these tips:

At fast-food restaurants:

- Choose a plain burger or cheeseburger, or a junior burger or cheeseburger.
- Choose a small serving of fries (or skip them entirely) or a baked potato.
- Choose apple wedges, another fruit, or carrot sticks as a side.
- Choose a salad with low-fat dressing on the side. Keep in mind that some salads can be huge portions or loaded with unhealthy ingredients. For those, order a half salad or read the nutritional information. You may want to skip some ingredients like chips or fried tacos.
- Choose grilled chicken and fish over fried foods.
- Order water or low-fat milk instead of soda.

At full-service restaurants:

- Choose grilled over fried items.
- Choose a baked potato or steamed vegetables over fries.
- Choose broth-based soups over cream soups.
- Ask your server if the chef could skip the salt on your entrée or vegetables (you can add it yourself if you like).
- Order salad with dressing on the side and no cheese.
- Order potatoes without gravy, butter, or sour cream. Eat plain, or top with steamed vegetables (another side) or salsa.
- Specify sautéed or steamed vegetables in place of creamy coleslaw.
- Choose a light or low-fat entrée.
- Order a turkey burger or veggie burger in place of a ground-beef burger.
- Order mini sliders versus a regular-size hamburger; eat two and bring one home to eat later.
- Eat half an entrée and bring the rest home, or share the entrée with a friend.

Make Like Choices

This is another important guideline, particularly when you are just starting out. It means to be aware of your substitutions and always try to substitute like foods. This translates into vegetables for vegetables or starchy foods for whole grains. To make things easier, whenever possible, try to substitute the same vegetable—like steamed broccoli with a sprinkle of almonds substituted for broccoli with cheese sauce, or brown rice substituted for white. There are several reasons for this. If you are just beginning the TLC diet, it will ensure that you like—and will eat—the foods you are choosing. There's no use substituting spinach for potato chips if you don't really like spinach. You'll end up not eating your veggie and, worse yet, wishing for the potato chips.

The second reason relates to portion sizes and satiety. Choose like foods so you won't be hungry. In an effort to jump in right away, some people go from eating a big cheeseburger to eating a small salad. This is the same thing as going from two slices of pizza to having one slice of toast with a tablespoon of peanut butter. This food will not fill you up, nor will it keep you satisfied.

Think about what food groups you are substituting from. Keep protein foods with protein foods. Perhaps replace a piece of pizza with a turkey sandwich on whole-wheat bread with mustard. Instead of eating a small salad alone, make a bigger salad and top it with a small amount of lean broiled steak or $^1/_2$ cup of cooked red or black beans. Save the peanut butter on toast for a snack, and instead make something more substantial, like a vegetable and tofu stir-fry. Experiment with foods you like to make the best choices.

Think About Taste and Texture

Many times we choose the foods we do because we like or want a certain taste or texture. The characteristics of a food—whether it's crunchy, creamy, salty, sweet, or savory—often directly relate to our desire for that food. Keep that in mind when you are making healthful substitutions. If you're craving something crunchy and salty, grabbing a bowl of grapes or strawberries is not going to make you happy. Instead, think about cutting up some carrot and celery sticks or having some brown rice cakes.

Be tuned in to what you really want and feel like having, and you won't be looking for more food later.

"Fat Free" Doesn't Always Mean Low Calorie

Not long ago, low-fat and fat-free foods were all the rage. Fueled by health recommendations that focused on fat, food manufacturers produced an avalanche of fat-free or low-fat desserts and sweets. Consumers were only too willing to buy them, splurging on these "fat-free" cookies, cakes, and ice cream with abandon.

What happened? Consumers who thought they couldn't get fat by eating fat-free cookies gained weight. But even worse than fostering our growing obesity epidemic, these foods can actually increase the risk of heart disease by raising triglyceride levels and lowering good HDL. By replacing the fats with sugars and refined carbohydrates, these foods actually did more harm than good. Furthermore, the calories in some brands were the same—and sometimes even more—than the regular brands.

Today fat-free and low-fat cookies, cakes, muffins, and other foods are not as popular as they once were, and the number of products has declined—but there are still plenty on the market. While I recommend low-fat or fat-free dairy products and crackers, most low-fat or fat-free sweet treats like cakes, cookies, and desserts are not worth having from a taste or health perspective. Many are loaded with artificial ingredients. If you do buy these products, think about portion control; even if it's low fat or fat free, it doesn't mean you can splurge. For example, many muffins are twice the size they were 20 years ago. Eat only half or a small portion, and save the rest for later (most times you can freeze it) or share it with a friend.

Think of these products as special treats, and make sure they are lower in calories than the original and/or low in calories in general. Pay attention to the serving size, and don't eat more than one serving at one time.

Tinkering with Recipes

Cutting the fat and salt in recipes can be a bit trickier than just removing or reducing the offending item. That's because salt, sugar, and fat do more than just add flavor. In baking, sugar contributes to tenderness and structure, keeps baked goods moist, and caramelizes during cooking, which enriches flavor and creates browning (it's also what gives breads a crisp crust).

Like sugar, fat tenderizes. It also affects texture and carries flavor. Solid fats, like butter, shortening, and margarine, are what make cakes light and airy: they hold air bubbles produced by leaveners. They are also responsible for the layers in pies and pastries, and they give cookies their spread.

Eggs provide color, flavor, texture, and richness to batters. The whites act as drying and leavening agents and add volume. The yolks are *emulsifiers*, meaning they bind fats with watery liquids and create a creamy consistency.

DEFINITION

An **emulsifier** is a substance that helps blend and stabilize a solution of oil- and water-based ingredients that would otherwise separate. Natural emulsifiers are egg yolks, peanuts, peanut butter, and cream.

Salt contributes to the overall flavor. In bread, it stops fermentation (so the bread doesn't rise too much) and strengthens the texture and protein of the bread.

Remember, anytime you change or substitute any ingredient in the recipe you are working with, you will get different results. Sometimes those changes will be so slight that most people won't notice them. Other times, you will create something unique and inspiring, fostering your imagination. Don't be afraid to experiment in the kitchen. Even if a change or substitution doesn't work, take it as a learning experience. Here are some guidelines that should help.

For Sugar

In many recipes, you can reduce the sugar by a quarter to a half the amount and add vanilla, nutmeg, or cinnamon to increase sweetness, without any real detrimental effects. Be aware that products with less sugar may have a different, more crumbly texture; may be drier; will have a shorter shelf life; and will be less brown than the original. Many times, as with cakes or breads that use vegetables like zucchini or sweet potatoes, this is not noticeable.

What kind of sugar you choose depends on the product. It also affects sweetness and texture. For example, honey is a liquid, so it adds moisture but it is not as sweet as table sugar. If you use it as a direct substitute (substitute honey for sugar in equal amounts) your product will taste different, but it will still give you the same amount of calories. Brown sugar, on the other hand, tastes sweeter than white sugar, so you might want to use less.

If you don't mind the aftertaste, artificial sweeteners are another option and can be used to cut sugar calories without cutting the sweetness. Many artificial sweeteners can now be used in baking. There are even some sugar and artificial sweetener blends that are specifically designed for baking; however, these are not calorie free.

For Fat

You can substitute 1 tablespoon of soft margarine (trans fat free) or $\frac{3}{4}$ tablespoon vegetable oil for 1 tablespoon of butter. In most recipes, you can substitute unsweetened applesauce, prune purée, mashed banana, or pumpkin butter for half the oil. You can also substitute cooking spray for fat used in frying or sautéing items.

For Dairy and Eggs

Dairy and eggs are other categories where you will find many high-fat and low-fat options. Choose the lower-fat options most of the time:

- Replace whole milk with nonfat or low-fat milk and 1 tablespoon vegetable oil.
- Replace heavy cream with evaporated skim milk or a combination of half low-fat yogurt and half plain, low-fat, unsalted cottage cheese.
- Replace sour cream with low-fat, unsalted cottage cheese blended with low-fat or nonfat yogurt, or use nonfat sour cream.
- Replace 8 ounces of cream cheese with 4 tablespoons soft margarine (trans fat free and low in saturated fat), blended with 1 cup low-fat, unsalted cottage cheese; add a small amount of fat-free milk, if necessary. See the list at the end of the chapter for other options.
- Replace eggs with two egg whites (for every one egg), or use a cholesterol-free egg substitute.

For Salt

Taking out the salt altogether usually isn't a good idea, as food will taste flat without it. But you can reduce it considerably. In most baking recipes, you can reduce the salt by half with no repercussions.

Some Smart Choices

The best way to make smart choices is to start with high-fat foods and then dial them down to make lower-fat choices. Though these foods may not always be considered low fat, they are better than their high-fat counterparts.

Instead of:	Substitute:
Fatty Meats	
Bacon and sausage	Canadian bacon, lean ham, turkey bacon, low-fat sausage, lean prosciutto
Fatty red meat	Loin or sirloin and round cuts, flank steak
Cold cuts or lunch meats	Low-fat and low-sodium cold cuts
Ground beef	93 percent lean, extra lean, or lean ground chicken or turkey breast, without the skin
Hot dogs	Low-fat all-natural turkey, chicken, or beef hot dogs
Dairy and Eggs	
Cream	Fat-free half and half, evaporated skim milk
Cream cheese	Low-fat or fat-free cream cheese, Neufchatel, or low-fat, unsalted cottage cheese, puréed until smooth
Cheese	Fat-free, low-fat, or reduced-fat cheese
Eggs	Two egg whites, or ¼ egg substitute (equal to one whole egg)
Sour cream	Nonfat or low-fat sour cream, or low-fat or nonfat yogurt, or a combination of half nonfat or low-fat yogurt and half low-fat, unsalted cottage cheese, puréed
Whole milk	Low-fat or fat-free milk, unsweetened soy milk, almond milk
Ice cream	Low-fat or fat-free ice cream or frozen yogurt, sherbets, frozen fruit bars
Custard and pudding	Pudding made with skim milk, applesauce
Yogurt, fruit flavored	Low-fat or fat-free plain yogurt, with added fresh fruit

Instead of:	Substitute:
Bread, Muffins, and Croissants	
White bread	Whole-grain breads with at least 4 grams fiber, 100 calories, and 170 milligrams sodium or less per slice
Croissants, brioches	Hard French rolls, Portuguese sweetbread, brown-'n'-serve rolls, and whole-wheat versions
Donuts, sweet rolls, muffins	Regular versions using unsaturated fat (oil or trans-fat-free margarine instead of butter)
	Low-fat options: English muffins, small bagel, reduced-fat or fat-free muffins or scones (beware of sugar)
Cake and pastries	Regular versions using unsaturated fat (oil or trans-fat-free margarine instead of butter)
	Low-fat options: Angel food cake, low-calorie fruit or nut breads, small or mini cupcakes with no frosting, mini (bite-size) pastries (using oil or trans-fat-free margarine)
Cookies	Regular versions using unsaturated fat (oil or trans-fat-free margarine instead of butter)
	Low-fat options: Reduced-fat or fat-free cookies (watch the sugar), graham crackers, ginger snaps or fig bars, vanilla wafers (compare calories)
White flour	In most recipes, can substitute half whole-wheat flour for white
Fried Foods and Snack Foods	
Fried foods	Grilled, baked, oven-fried, or broiled foods
Potato chips and corn chips	Baked potato chips (buy low-sodium brands)
Tortilla chips	Baked tortilla chips, whole-wheat crackers, or rice cakes
Chocolate	Cocoa (mostly used in baking or drinking) or dark chocolate, 60 percent or more
Extras	
Salt	Herbs and spices, salt-free seasonings, citrus peel, garlic powder, onion powder
Butter, shortening	Trans-fat-free soft margarines, vegetable oil, low-saturated fat, reduced-fat, or low-fat butter

Once you get the hang of it, making healthy substitutions is fast and easy. All it takes is a little time and practice.

The Least You Need to Know

- When making healthy substitutions, choose foods that you like and that are comparable to higher-fat items.
- Low-fat and fat-free foods are not always the best choice because they can be high in sugar and calories.
- Healthy substitutions will shave off fat and calories and generally will not affect the finished product.
- The main nutrients to consider when determining whether you want to make a substitution are saturated fat, cholesterol, sugar, salt, and calories.

Maintaining Success Away from Home

Chapter 12

In This Chapter

- Tips for eating out wisely
- What to do with oversize portions
- How to handle social functions
- Secrets of a heart-healthy eater

Just because you're on the TLC diet doesn't mean you have to give up eating out or eating with friends. That's good news because many of us dine out frequently. In fact, the average American spends nearly half (about 48 percent) of each food dollar away from home. Unfortunately, most restaurant foods are loaded with fat, salt, and calories.

For this reason, you shouldn't make a habit of dining in restaurants, but you can enjoy occasional outings as special treats—the way it used to be—as long as you keep a few things in mind. In this chapter, I tell you what you need to know to make dining out easy and heart healthy, without breaking the bank or stressing yourself out.

Eating at someone's house or at parties or picnics also poses some concerns for people who are watching their diet. But don't let this stand in your way of socializing. You can take plenty of actions to put your host at ease and have a good time while still following your TLC diet.

Remember, we live in a country where quality, nutritious food is all around us. It's just a matter of making the right choices to find it. And that's actually easier than you think.

Choose Wisely

The first step in going to a restaurant is finding the right one. That's one that offers healthful, low-saturated-fat, low-cholesterol options, without going overboard on salt and calories, that still taste good! Considering that, according to the National Restaurant Association, there are more than 970 million food service establishments in the United States, you'd think it would be easy to find one that fits these criteria. It's not.

According to the USDA's Economic Research Service, people who eat out often have poorer diets than those who eat more foods at home. Diners eat fewer vegetables, fruits, whole grains, and dairy, along with more saturated fat, calories, sodium, and added sugars than those who prepare food at home. About a third of our calories come from restaurant or take-out food.

Despite the fact that many restaurants have added menu items with health and taste in mind, the numbers don't always add up. This means many items are still high in saturated fat, calories, and sodium. The good news is, it's easy for you to figure out whether a restaurant is right for you. That's because a fair number of food service establishments now provide nutrition information to their customers either online or at the store.

GOTCHA!

A 2012 report from the Rand Corporation analyzed more than 30,000 menu entrées from 245 chain restaurants and found that 96 percent of entrées exceeded daily recommendations for calories, fat, sodium, and saturated fat. Among the interesting findings: family-style restaurants fared worse than fast-food restaurants, and appetizers averaged 130 calories higher than entrées.

Much of this disclosure is thanks to 2010 legislation that requires chain restaurants with 20 or more locations (along with bakeries, grocery stores, convenience stores, and grocery chains) to provide nutrition information for each of their menu items. Although as of May 2012 final regulations regarding exact requirements are still pending, some of the industry has already jumped on the bandwagon.

For people concerned about their health and their heart, like those on the TLC plan, knowing these numbers is essential for sticking to your diet plan and deciding what restaurant to choose. Here are a few other things to consider when deciding where to go.

Avoid Fast Food

Fast food is quick, convenient, and cheap. It's also readily available (or so it seems) on practically every corner. But it comes with a price. Eating too much and eating it on a regular basis takes a toll on our health. Science now points to fast food as a major contributor to our rising rates of obesity, diabetes, high blood pressure, and heart disease.

From a nutritional standpoint, fast food is high in calories, saturated fat, cholesterol, and sodium, and it lacks fiber, minerals, and several vitamins. Although it is possible to make better choices (see Chapter 11), there are drawbacks. First, the menu is limited, with few or no vegetables. Second, the food is highly processed and has a lot of calories for little nutrients. Third, special requests are not really an option because most of the food is premade.

HEALTHFUL LIVING

In July 2011, the National Restaurant Association launched the Kids LiveWell program, a national restaurant program designed to offer kids healthful offerings that meet nutrition criteria based on leading health organizations recommendations and the USDA Dietary Guidelines. The initiative now includes some 95 restaurants in 25,000 locations.

Go Online and Use Social Media

Checking out the restaurant online is a *must* before you even step out the door. Nearly all restaurants now post their menus online. If they don't, plenty of other places, like Yelp (yelp.com), Urban Spoon (urbanspoon.com), and Zagat (zagat.com), can give you an idea of what restaurants offer. You can also do an online search for a restaurant and see what happens. Once you do find a menu, open it and read it. Be aware that sometimes restaurants have separate menus for their lighter fare that may not be online. If after that you don't see anything that you think is appropriate, skip the restaurant and try another.

Nutrition information may be listed on the menu, on a separate page on the restaurant's website, or in print only at the restaurant. Chain restaurants, in particular, usually do a good job of providing this information in innovative ways. Some have even created special health-oriented programs. For example, Burgerville, a chain that is based in the Northwest, gives personalized nutrition information for each item on receipts. Each receipt lists calories, protein, carbohydrates, and fat for the meal, along with percentages of this breakdown based on a 2,000- and 2,500-calorie meal.

Other places, like Au Bon Pain, have come up with a "smart menu" concept that allows you to search menu items online based on the lowest amount of saturated fat, calories, sodium, carbohydrates, and cholesterol. You can also find the highest-fiber items in each category.

At its restaurants, Silver Diner, an East Coast chain, highlights healthful, locally produced meals under its Eat Well Do Well program right on the menu. All menu items are promoted as having 600 calories or less, and the menu lists fat, saturated fat, cholesterol, and fiber below each item. Every heart-healthy dish is noted with a red heart. Consider these other examples of chain restaurants that offer better-for-you menu items and easy-to-read nutrition information:

Fast Casual	Casual Restaurants
Panera Bread	Uno Chicago Grill
Jason's Deli	Souplantation and Sweet Tomatoes (two chains)
Au Bon Pain	Mimi's Café (Lifestyle menu)
Noodles and Company	PF Chang's China Bistro
Corner Bakery	Bob Evans (Fit from the Farm)
Chipotle	Ruby Tuesday
Atlanta Bread	Romano's Macaroni Grill (Sensible Fare)
McDonald's	Chevy's Fresh Mex
Einstein Bros. Bagels	Olive Garden (Garden Fare)
Taco Del Mar	Denny's (Fit-Fare)

Based on an article by Health *magazine (look for it at Health.com, "America's Healthiest"). For fast casual, an expert panel reviewed the 100 largest quick-service chains; for casual restaurants, the expert panel looked at 96 fast-service and sit-down restaurants.*

If you find an item you like, be sure to check out the nutritional information on it first—you might change your mind. Saturated fat is likely to be in check, but sodium levels can go through the roof.

If you're not sure where you want to go or whether you need help figuring out the right restaurant, try searching at healthydiningfinder.com. This site offers dietitian-approved menu items and nutrition information for local restaurants. You can also find apps that do the same thing, like the Food Tracker Healthy Dining Out app.

Another option is to take advantage of social media. Look at the restaurant's Facebook page. Follow it on Twitter. See what people are saying about it. This may also be another way to find out about other restaurants that offer more healthful options either at home or in other cities. If you are traveling for business, social media can help you find heart-friendly restaurants out of town.

Look to Ethnic Restaurants

Many reasons support visiting an ethnic restaurant over a more traditional "American" one. It is easier to find vegetarian and vegan menu items. Indian cuisine is well known for the wide variety of vegetarian dishes and meat used as a condiment. This is also true in Chinese, Japanese, Thai, and other Asian cuisines. Think about adding vegetables to rice or noodle dishes.

Since this cuisine is usually made to order, it also may be a bit easier (depending on the restaurant) for you to make changes or special requests. Finally, ethnic cooking tends to utilize more vegetables as side dishes or in mixed dishes. For example, Chinese restaurants generally use a wide variety of cooking greens, not just spinach.

HEART-SMART HABITS

Many Chinese restaurants now offer steamed vegetables upon request. Make your own main dish by combining an order of fried rice or seasoned noodles with an order of steamed vegetables, and you've got an instant easy meal.

Small mom-and-pop ethnic restaurants have one drawback. Under the new law, they are not required to provide nutrition information, so they don't. Consequently, it's harder to find out whether a meal fits your criteria. Since many of these dishes use a large number of ingredients, some of which may be exclusive to the cuisine and hard to find, deciphering ingredient information can be a challenge. However, you are more likely able to strike up a relationship with the owner in these places; he or she may be able to address any health concerns you have.

What to Order

Once you've decided where to go, it's time to look at the menu and pick what to order. If the restaurant has a "light" or "healthy" menu program, choose from that. Other times, dishes may be tagged with a special symbol or bullet. In any case, it's good to look at nutritional information, since sometimes healthy menu items are not as healthy as they seem.

If the food service establishment doesn't have any special items, never fear—you can still learn to maneuver through the menu on your own. Here are a few tips to help you make smart choices.

Skip the Sauce

Many restaurant meals are dressed with some kind of sauce. This can be BBQ sauce, butter sauce, cream sauce, cheese sauce, "special house" sauce, ranch dressing, honey mustard, mayonnaise—the list goes on and on. Many of these items are convenience foods, bought already prepared.

On menus, they are considered a value-added item that often bumps up price. They're also generally high in fat, saturated fat, salt, and sugar. Your best bet is to skip the sauce altogether and eat the dish plain. If that's not your style choose a healthier sauce, like ketchup or mustard. If you really want the sauce the restaurant offers, ask for it on the side and use only half. Typical restaurant meals load on sauces, often pouring on more than most people would add themselves.

Steer Clear of Meat and Cheese

One of the biggest adjustments on the TLC diet is learning to eat less meat and cheese. This is easier at home—but when it comes to dining out, things get more challenging. Food service operations are notorious for loading on protein portions like meat, chicken, and fish. Sandwiches boasting 10 ounces of turkey, steaks weighing 16 ounces or more, and half-pound burgers are the norm.

The amount of cheese piled on food can be just as extreme. Consider quesadillas, alfredo sauces, and cheesy fries, not to mention the cheese that adorns everything from sandwiches and burgers to burritos and nachos. And, of course, there's pizza. Do yourself a favor and skip the cheese and the meat altogether. Instead, focus on vegan options, like bean and rice burritos, grilled vegetable sandwiches without the cheese, and Asian-oriented stir-fry. Just beware of sodium.

If you do order a protein, go for skinless, boneless chicken breast or fish—then only eat half and take home the rest.

Forget Fried

Fried foods are not a good pick on the TLC diet. In addition to the extra fat and calories fried foods have, the oil restaurants use to fry food can be high in trans fats—the worst kind of fat. Some less expensive oils, like palm and coconut oil, are also high in saturated fat.

Finally, the type of food you'll find breaded and fried isn't exactly health food. Occasionally, you can find fried breaded green beans, zucchini, mushrooms, or even broccoli, but usually the options are less healthy. More familiar fare is fried chicken wings, fried cheese, fried meat dumplings, and fried egg rolls or spring rolls. Since fried foods are particularly prevalent on appetizer menus, your best bet is to skip the opening course and order something baked, grilled, or broiled instead.

Beware of Portion Distortion

Over the years, portion sizes in restaurant have ballooned to double and sometimes triple what they were just 30 years ago. The worst part is that many of us don't even realize it. A slew of media coverage, along with a push by consumer watchdog organizations like Center for Science in the Public Interest (cspinet.org), has brought attention to the issue and forced some restaurant to act. Consequently, several restaurants now offer half sandwiches and soup or salad, "shareable" appetizers, and regular and small sizes. Some even allow adults to buy a kids' menu option. Following are some tips on what to do if a restaurant doesn't have downsize programs in place.

Order an Appetizer for Dinner

In many restaurants, appetizer portions are big enough to be an entrée of their own. Instead of buying from the main dish section, consider ordering off the appetizer menu. Then let the waiter or waitress know that you want the appetizer served with the main entrées. This works well when there is a long list of a variety of appetizer items to choose from.

HEALTHFUL LIVING

According to the National Restaurant Association's 2012 chef survey, the top two appetizer trends are vegetarian and vegetable appetizers and ethnic, street-food appetizers like kabobs and hummus.

Since chefs offer appetizers in smaller portions, items in this section of the menu tend to be a bit more creative and adventuresome. If you're the type of person who likes to try new foods, ordering off the appetizer menu may be a real treat and offer you the opportunity to try something you wouldn't normally try.

Share with Someone

After years of dining out, I rarely order a full entrée just for myself. I've learned that portions are way too big and that I just don't have the willpower to stop eating. Instead, I split an entrée with my dining companion, and both of us leave happy and full, but not stuffed.

Over the years, I have noticed restaurants become more accommodating to this type of dining. In fact, at one of my favorite spots, the waitress divides the portion before it even gets to the table and serves us individually. In this case, you don't even feel like you're sharing, and the portions are just right.

Sharing allows you to split the portion as well as the bill, saving you money and calories. It also may allow you to order another item. My husband and I usually split a small salad and order an entrée. The hardest part is deciding on a meal that both you and your partner want. Once you've gotten over that hurdle, the rest is a piece of cake.

Take It Home

If you don't want to split an order but the entrée is too large for you, consider boxing up half as soon as your entrée reaches the table. If you do this before you start eating (ask the waiter or waitress to bring you a take-out container when she brings your meal), you won't be tempted to overeat. This also ensures that you have a meal for lunch or dinner the next day. It's a win-win situation all around.

Make Special Requests

Don't be afraid to make special requests. This is your most important tool for eating the TLC way. Your server is your lifeline to the kitchen. Explain what you are looking for and what you want to avoid. Then ask for suggestions. Your server should also be able to explain what is in every dish and how it is prepared. If your server can't, ask him or her to check with the chef and let you know.

Once you know what you want, ask the server if you can make some changes. Usually this involves skipping the sauce, upping the vegetables, and substituting fries for a baked potato or brown rice. Keep in mind that the more changes you make, the more likely it will be that the kitchen makes mistakes. Try to find dishes on the menu that need only a few changes.

Sometimes restaurants will even have build-your-own salads, sandwiches, or entrées featuring several items you can choose from.

Parties, Get-Togethers, and Social Occasions

Not every occasion to eat out is at a restaurant. Picnics, barbecues, and holiday parties are other times you will be dining out. So how do you stick to your TLC diet when you're at these events?

Bring Your Own

You should have no trouble eating a cholesterol-lowering diet at a potluck picnic. Why? For one thing, you'll be bringing your own dish to share. Choose something that is substantial enough to be a meal if there are no other healthy choices. This is also an opportunity to show your friends how delicious heart-healthy food can be.

What happens when you're not sure whether you should bring something? Call the host and ask. Start out by saying, "May I bring something to the party so you don't have to fuss?" This also takes the pressure off the host of having to prepare a "special" meal for you.

Another approach, especially for a barbecue, is to offer to bring some vegetables that could just be thrown on the grill. Be sure to have them already cut and prepped with a favorite spice and a sprinkle of olive oil. Tossed with a small amount of grilled chicken, fish, or steak and some greens, this makes a simple, satisfying meal at any party.

Holiday Parties

Holiday parties can be a minefield of high-fat, high-calorie foods that can wreak havoc with your diet, even if you have the best intentions. To keep yourself from losing self-control and still have a good time, follow these simple steps.

Have a healthful snack before you go. Carrot sticks, some fruit, and a cup of yogurt are good choices. This takes the edge off your hunger and prevents you from making a beeline for the food table as soon as you walk in the door. It also means you'll be more inclined to make better food choices. Many people skip meals when they know they are going to a party at night, hoping to "save up" calories. Don't fall into this trap. If you're hungry, you're more likely to make poor food choices. Eat light before you go and think about the food you take.

Take a taste. Holidays are a time when rich, luscious food abounds. This may be the only time certain foods are made or offered. Don't deprive yourself of special treats, but don't go overboard, either. Be sure it's something worth the extra calories, and take only one or two bites.

> **HEART-SMART HABITS**
>
> Giving in to cravings now and then is key to having a successful, healthful meal plan. Studies show dieters who occasionally give in to cravings are more likely to stay on their diet and lose weight than those who don't give in.

Talk more, eat less. Since holiday parties are often social events where people get together with friends and colleagues, it's easy to eat without thinking. Mindless eating, which I talk more about in Chapter 13, means eating without thinking and often leads to overeating and poor food choices. This is easy to do when you're busy socializing. To avoid this trap, put only a few things on your plate and walk away from the table. This allows you to socialize without overeating.

On the opposite side of the coin, when you're at a party and know few people, resist the urge to find your comfort zone near the food table. Instead, force yourself to walk away from the table and meet new people. Talking will also prevent you from eating more.

Learning the Tricks of the Trade

Eating a heart-smart TLC diet isn't hard to do, but it does require being a more conscious eater. This means paying attention to the quality and quantity of food you eat. With a little practice, you'll learn to do this without even thinking about it. Holiday parties need a bit more vigilance because people are more relaxed and the food is more likely to be richer than usual. If you follow these four tips, you're sure to make it through.

Scope out the buffet before you eat. Walk around the buffet before you get in line. Make a mental note of what foods are good choices and what foods are not. Then decide (from the good choices) what you want, based on what you'd like to eat. Typically, buffets are designed to have the inexpensive foods, like vegetables and starches, first and the more expensive foods, like proteins, last. You want to fill half your plate with fruits and vegetables (that includes green salads), a quarter of your plate with starches, and a quarter or less with protein.

Go veggie. Home in on seasonal produce. Nearly all holiday parties have a crudité or raw vegetable platter. Skip the dip, or take only a small amount, and fill up on these veggies. Roasted vegetables are another good option. Pick plainer vegetables, such as green beans almondine over green bean casserole, and don't be afraid to take several "side" vegetables on your plate.

Small plates, small bites. If your eyes are bigger than your stomach, rein in portion sizes by using a salad plate or small dinner plate rather than the typical oversize plates many hotel catering operations offer. By loading up a small plate, you will feel satisfied without feeling deprived. You'll also fit less on your plate so you won't overeat—just don't go up for seconds.

Start with water. Many people forget to count the fact that alcohol has calories. Drinking too much can also lead you to overeat and eat the wrong foods. When you first arrive, particularly if you haven't eaten in a while, be sure to drink a glass of water before you have a glass of wine. Once you've got some food in your stomach, you can imbibe. To stretch your drink calories, try adding a splash of seltzer to your wine for a wine spritzer.

GOTCHA!

Regardless of whether they contain alcohol, some holiday drinks are high in saturated fat and filled with sugar. Two classic holiday beverages fall into this category: holiday eggnog and rich hot chocolate laced with heavy cream. These sugar-sweetened beverages are off limits on the TLC diet, but if you must have a taste, take a sip or two and leave the rest.

Managing your TLC diet when you're dining out, eating out of town, or noshing at holiday parties isn't as easy as eating at home, but it is possible with a little bit of work and planning.

The Least You Need to Know

- It's possible to eat out on the TLC diet, but it requires vigilance and extra effort.
- Choosing the right restaurant means checking out the menu and, if possible, nutrition information before you go.
- People on the TLC diet should gravitate toward vegan or vegetarian items on restaurant menus and make special requests to remove fatty sauces.

- Holiday parties don't have to be off-limits. Be prepared by eating a small snack before you go, checking out the food before you eat, and drinking a glass of water first.
- At buffets, home in on plain vegetables, fruits, and whole grains, and avoid cheese, rich sauces, fried foods, and high-fat proteins.

Chapter 13

Learning a New Lifestyle

In This Chapter

- Changing bad eating habits
- Enjoying the benefits of exercise
- Destressing your life
- Getting sleep for your heart

When it comes to improving heart health, more matters than what you eat. When and how you eat—along with other factors like stress, physical activity, and sleep—makes a difference. In other words, it's your entire lifestyle.

Indeed, lifestyle factors have a huge impact on our eating behavior and, ultimately, our health. And this part of our life often needs a major overhaul when it comes to feeling fit and strong.

In the United States, the demands of modern society take a big toll on our health. Time-crunched Americans get little exercise, lack sleep, and are chronically stressed. This leads to overeating, mindless eating, and eating on the run, not to mention poor food choices. Since bad habits foster more bad habits, this creates a vicious cycle.

But if you want to stay healthy, you've got to learn to break these bad habits and replace them with good ones. Here I discuss how external cues like our environment influence our eating habits and affect our health. Then I give you ways to help take control of your life, one step at a time.

Granted, making lifestyle changes doesn't happen overnight, but it isn't as hard as you think. Sometimes all it takes is one or two changes to feel and see a difference. These positive changes then motivate you to do more, and before you know it, you're leading a healthier, happier, and less stressful life.

Breaking Bad Habits

Many of us fall into bad habits not by choice, but by chance. Dictated by time, convenience, work schedules, and other aspects of life, they eventually become part of our routine. We don't think about them. But that doesn't mean we can't change them. Some habits are easy to break; others take a bit more time and effort. The key to success involves three steps:

1. **Become conscious of your habit.** A habit becomes a habit, good or bad, precisely because we don't think about it. We do it without thinking. This then becomes part of our routine. Think about what you're doing and when, why you have fallen into this habit, and how it makes you feel, and you'll be more likely to change it.
2. **Write it down.** Write down exactly what kind of change you want. This could be a habit you want to break or a habit you want to start. For example: *I want to exercise 30 minutes every day* or *I want to stop eating in front of the television.* Writing down the habit you want to achieve or change makes it a clear, more concrete goal. Make your habit as simple as possible.
3. **Replace your bad habit with a good one.** This means changing the offending behavior or creating a new habit. Whether this is going to the gym every day at lunch or counting to 10 before you get angry, some kind of conscious effort is involved to do something different. Eventually, you want the habit to become automatic, like brushing your teeth in the morning or combing your hair. This requires the habit to be relatively easy to do and produce positive feedback—rewards. Remember, it also takes time.

HEALTHFUL LIVING

Chances are, the longer you've had a habit, the longer it will take to break it. While it is almost impossible to pinpoint a time, some experts say that after 30 days of changing your habits, it gets easier but you can still be derailed. After a year, however, not doing the habit is harder than doing it.

When it comes to making healthful food choices, the best advice is to make these healthful foods as easy as possible, while making unhealthful choices hard. As humans, we will always follow the path of least resistance. Therefore, if you put junk food in the back of the closet or on the top shelf where it's impossible to reach (or better yet, don't buy it at all) and put fresh veggies on the table already cut up or have fruit washed and ready to eat in the front of the refrigerator, chances are you will go for the veggies and fruit. Do this on a regular basis for a month, and eating these foods will be like second nature. Following are four good habits you want to incorporate into your everyday TLC diet.

Make Time for Meals

This includes breakfast, lunch, and dinner. All too often, people become overwhelmed with everyday commitments, and the first thing to slide is their meals. This is particularly true with breakfast, the most-skipped meal—and also the most important meal of the day.

If you find yourself eating on the run, eating in the car, or skipping meals on a regular basis, you need to re-evaluate your schedule and make a change. Eating this way is bad for you and your health in more ways than one.

It affects digestion and absorption, meaning that you can't process your food at optimal levels. It's not good for your heart. The grab-and-go foods you're likely to eat in this lifestyle are overly processed, overly salty, and laden with unhealthful saturated fat, cholesterol, and calories—exactly the type of foods you should avoid on the TLC diet. This pattern also makes you more likely to overeat. Since portion sizes in convenience foods have more than doubled in the last 20 years, it's more likely that the bag of chips or bottled drink you bought contains two or three servings rather than one. Finally, wolfing down your meal in a few seconds flat is just not a good way to enjoy your food.

HEART-SMART HABITS

Have breakfast every morning. After a good night's sleep and several hours of fasting, a healthful breakfast provides the energy you need to jump-start your day and stay alert. A good breakfast includes low-fat protein, whole grains, fruits, and/or vegetables. (For breakfast recipe ideas, check out Chapter 15.)

Being too busy to eat a healthful, balanced meal is not an option on the TLC diet. Spend time preparing nutritious foods that you like, and then spend time eating them. In return, you will nourish your body and your mind. Share these meals with the people you love, and you'll build better, stronger relationships as well.

Become a Mindful Eater

How many times have you plowed through a large meal without even remembering a single bite? This is mindless eating. It's eating with no regard to the food we're putting into our mouths and with no regard to what our body needs or wants. It allows us to consume hundreds of calories above and beyond what we need at the moment and not enjoy a single bite.

Of all the ways people have become mindless eaters—eating while working, eating while reading, eating while playing on the computer—eating while watching television is the most common. It's also the most harmful. Not only do you not pay attention to what you eat, but the commercials encourage you to eat high-calorie, fatty foods. And the long programs (half-hour to hour shows or longer) mean you can eat mindlessly for long periods of time.

To become a mindful eater is to pay attention to your food and the act of eating. This means eating with all five senses, learning what you like and don't like, and listening to your body, which will tell you when you're full. It means sitting down at the table to a meal that you eat slowly and purposely.

What will be your reward? Eating will become a pleasure to be savored and enjoyed. You'll appreciate (even more) eating the healthful foods that fill your plate and being in tune with your body. You'll ultimately eat less, and you won't even know it!

Switch to Water

Most beverages we drink are of the sugar-sweetened variety—sodas, energy drinks, sports drinks, sweetened tea. Many of these we drink without thinking and without compensating for their calories.

One of the easiest habits to get used to is drinking water in place of these beverages. To make things easier, get rid of all the sugar-sweetened drinks at home or in the office. In their place, put bottles of water. Keep them icy cold and always filled to the brim. Not only will water keep you hydrated, but it will also make you feel full, thus curbing your appetite.

Don't Snack Late at Night

It's not a good idea to eat late at night or anytime after dinner (around 7 or 8 P.M.). Nighttime snacking usually involves high-calorie, fatty foods, like fast food, pizza, and potato chips—foods you shouldn't have on the TLC diet. In one 2011 study from Northwestern University, people who went to bed late ate twice as much fast food and half as many fruits and vegetables as those with earlier bedtimes. They were also more likely to drink full-calorie sodas and eat more total calories in a day. Consequently, subjects who went to bed late and ate late at night weighed more than those who went to bed earlier.

Poor food choices and increased calories aren't the only ways we can put on the pounds if we eat late at night. Animal studies show that mice that ate around the clock gained more weight and had a poorer metabolic profile than mice that ate during the day, even though they ate the same number of calories.

HEALTHFUL LIVING

Shift workers who eat late at night tend to be more overweight and have poorer health than those who don't work at night.

What to do? Make it a point to stop eating after dinner. If you must nibble on something, make sure it is a healthful snack that includes protein, carbohydrates, and a small amount of fat and contains no more than 200 calories, like low-fat cheese or nuts. Also be sure to stop eating at least two hours before bedtime, to give your body a chance to digest the food.

Exercise: A Heart-Smart Habit

There's no question that exercise is essential for good health. The benefits of exercise can't be emphasized enough. It strengthens the heart, increases muscle mass, builds strong bones, helps in weight management, decreases stress, enhances cognitive function, and improves overall health. Yet it's something many of us just don't do enough of. Only half of Americans report exercising for at least 30 minutes a day three days a week, and about 33 percent of Americans don't get any exercise.

From a cardiovascular perspective, regular physical activity improves circulation, lowers blood pressure, reduces LDL cholesterol, raises HDL cholesterol, and lowers triglycerides. It also helps control diabetes. Consequently, being physically active on a regular basis is a key part of the TLC program.

Aerobic activity is the best type of exercise for your heart because it dilates the blood vessels and improves circulation (among many other benefits). And vigorous exercise is better than moderate or light exercise. But even low-intensity exercise is better than nothing. While clinical trials have found as much as a 60 percent reduction in heart disease risk, depending on intensity and duration of exercise, the general consensus is that physical activity lowers risk of cardiovascular disease by 20 to 30 percent.

To get these benefits, experts recommend 30 minutes of moderate-intensity exercise every day, or at least five days a week (that amounts to $2^1/_2$ hours a week). This includes activities like brisk walking, biking, jogging, or swimming. You don't have to do it all at once, either; you can break it up into shorter 10-minute intervals.

But when it comes to exercise, more is better. Researchers found that when exercisers increased their activity from 30 minutes to 60 minutes a period (totaling 300 minutes a week, or 5 hours a week), benefits were greater.

This doesn't mean you should jump into exercising right away, particularly if you've been sedentary. Overdoing it can do more harm than good, increasing your risk of injury and actually harming your heart. Always check with your doctor before you start any exercise program, particularly if you have heart disease or high blood pressure, or if you are a man over 40 or a woman over 50 who has not exercised in recent years.

The Hazards of Sitting

With the rise of computers and a lifestyle centered on watching rather than doing, the latest research has focused on a specific type of sedentary behavior: the dangers of too much sitting. It has shown that prolonged sitting for six or more hours a day significantly increases your risk of cardiovascular disease and shortens your life. Just consider the amount of time spent sitting at your desk, at your computer, and in your car.

Then tack on "recreational sitting," like sitting for entertainment—watching TV shows and movies and playing computer games. A 2011 study found that people who spend four hours or more on this type of screen-based entertainment are twice as likely to have a cardiac event like a heart attack than those who spend less than two hours each day. This same study also found that people who sat longer had an almost 50 percent greater risk of dying from any cause than those who sat for less time.

Research also shows that sitting may be worse for women than for men, for both heart disease and diabetes. Women who sat for longer periods of time were at greater risk of developing type 2 diabetes.

What else has the new research uncovered about prolonged sitting?

- People who sit for prolonged periods of time have a bigger belly than those who don't.
- People with sitting jobs have twice the rate of cardiovascular disease as people with standing or walking jobs.
- Prolonged sitting lowers HDL cholesterol.
- Sitting for long periods results in less healthy measures of triglycerides, insulin, and insulin resistance.
- Prolonged sitting reduces the rate at which you burn calories.
- People who sit for prolonged periods have lowered life expectancy from all causes of death.

HEART-SMART HABITS

If you're sitting at your desk for long periods of time, be sure to take short breaks and get up every hour. This can make a difference in protecting heart health.

The good news is, you can do something about it, even if you have a desk job or spend a lot of time in the car. The solution: get up. Research shows that getting up and moving around for even just a few minutes periodically (every hour) can undo some of the damage of prolonged sitting. Another option is to stretch and twist in your seat. Even if you just stand for a few minutes, that's better than nothing.

Stress Less

Although we don't know exactly how, we do know that stress increases the risk of heart disease. Two types of stress exist: chronic emotional stress, which is the stress of everyday life, and the stress that is most likely to take its toll on our health; and intense or acute stress, which can be either physical or emotional. This is the stress that comes on quickly, usually from a traumatic event, and causes the heart to race, blood pressure to rise (temporarily), and veins to constrict.

Chronic emotional stress makes you more likely to develop atherosclerosis. Intense stress can lead to an acute heart problem, such as a heart attack. Both types of stress signal the brain to tell the adrenal gland to release adrenalin and cortisol, two fight-or-flight hormones that cause metabolic changes that can worsen vascular function.

But chronic stress does more damage because it keeps these hormones at persistently high levels, resulting in vascular harm over time and also increasing inflammation.

Indirectly, chronic stress increases your chances of developing other major risk factors of heart disease, such as obesity, because it can lead to overeating.

Stress can be particularly harmful to people with *Type A personalities*. Early studies linking heart disease to Type A's found that one of every two men is likely to be a Type A personality. These studies also show that men with Type A personalities are twice as likely to have heart disease than those who are not Type A. Recently, science has questioned this conclusion, but characteristics of Type A's still can lead to heart disease.

Luckily, not everyone responds to stress in the same way. Some people cope better than others. Coping refers to your thoughts and behavior in response to the perception of stress. Coping seeks to lessen the negative effects of what's bothering you.

DEFINITION

In general, people with **Type A personalities** are always in a hurry; quick to be irritable, impatient, or angry; and are perfectionists.

Everyone gets stressed out once in a while; it's how you deal with stress that matters. Each of us has a unique set of stressors and a unique way of dealing with stress. The best way to minimize stress is to catch it in the early stages. Identify your stressors and work from there. How you deal with stress depends on the stressor. Here are a few general tips:

- **Improve your time-management techniques.** Much of our stress revolves around not having enough time in the day to manage all we want to do. Re-evaluate your priorities and set realistic goals. Then block out specific times to accomplish your tasks.
- **Follow the TLC diet.** When you're stressed, diet tends to fall by the wayside. Yet this is the time you most need to follow a healthful diet. Eating plenty of healthful fruits and vegetables actually keeps you strong so you can better handle stress.
- **Learn mental relaxation strategies.** Mental relaxation strategies allow you to accept what you cannot change. This includes meditation, yoga, relaxation rituals like taking a bath or going for a walk, and guided imagery (generating positive images in your mind).

- **Exercise.** Exercise, particularly vigorous exercise, is an amazing stress reducer. Not only does it physically help you relieve tension, but it mentally requires focus and complete attention. This takes your mind off the stress and helps you refocus.

Learning better stress-management skills takes time, patience, and practice. It involves learning a better way to respond to stress. This means finding constructive ways to let go of the things you can't change and solving or changing the things you can. In this book, I just scratch the surface of what stress management involves. If you want to learn a new approach to stress management and find out more, consider getting a book on the subject. You can find many good ones online or at the bookstore. Pick what works best for you.

Sleep on It

In our society where cellphones, email, Twitter, and Facebook make instant communication a 24-hour necessity, sleep is a hot commodity. It's also essential for good health. Although sleep patterns differ over time and from person to person, humans optimally need from seven to eight hours of sleep each night to thrive.

Too little sleep—six hours or less—increases your risk of stroke, heart attack, and congestive heart failure. Based on a survey of more than 3,000 adults who participated in the National Health and Nutrition Examination Survey (NHANES), people consistently getting less than six hours of sleep were 2 times more likely to have a stroke or heart attack and 1.6 times more likely to get congestive heart failure. Other studies have linked too little sleep with greater likelihood of insulin resistance and type 2 diabetes.

People who sleep less are also more likely to be overweight or obese, which leads to other health issues. Why? People who are tired tend to make poor food choices, like eating junk food. Spending more time awake also might mean they have more time to eat, and being tired means less energy to burn. Lately, scientists have found another reason sleep can put on the pounds: it throws off your body's natural hormone balance for eating. People who are deprived of sleep have higher levels of ghrelin, a hunger hormone that stimulates appetite, and lower levels of leptin, which tells the brain that the body is full. Furthermore, these hormonal levels stay out of whack for a full day after your long night.

HEALTHFUL LIVING

Getting too much sleep—nine hours or more a night—also has its problems. Oversleeping has been linked to increased risk of heart disease, diabetes, and death. While making up for lost sleep with a long bout in bed is okay, researchers think regularly oversleeping may be a sign of a sleep disorder or other underlying condition, such as depression.

As we age, getting a good night's sleep gets harder, mostly because our sleep wave patterns change. But that's okay because older adults (over 60 years of age) are better able to cope with sleep deprivation than younger adults. What's the best way to ensure a good night's sleep? Exercise regularly, eat a healthful TLC diet, and keep a handle on stress and anxiety. Some people swear by a warm bath or low-intensity yoga. If it works for you, go for it.

Making lifestyle changes is not always easy, but once you start, you'll be motivated by feeling and looking good.

The Least You Need to Know

- Break bad eating habits by consciously replacing them with positive behaviors that promote a healthful lifestyle.
- To prevent mindless eating, overeating, and skipping meals, pay attention to when, what, and where you eat. Be sure to make time for every meal.
- Regular exercise for 30 minutes at least five times a week is essential for good heart health.
- Reduce stress by managing your time, practicing relaxation techniques, and following the TLC diet.
- To feel your best and have optimum health, get seven to eight hours of sleep every night.

Chapter 14

What to Do If It's Not Working

In This Chapter

- Send in the superfoods
- Consider more fiber
- Eat more plant foods
- Enjoy more seafood
- Track your progress in a food journal

Researchers estimate that decreasing saturated fat in your diet can reduce LDL cholesterol by 8 to 10 percent. But not everyone responds the same way to diet and exercise changes, and not everyone follows the diet the same way. Furthermore, some foods are better than others at lowering cholesterol. Consequently, if your doctor thinks you're not making as much progress as you should, or if you just want to give your health and your cholesterol levels a jump-start, you can eat certain foods to sweep away bad cholesterol and make more good cholesterol.

These are the superfoods of heart health because they are known to effectively lower LDL cholesterol without hurting HDL cholesterol. They include certain plant foods, foods high in fiber, and some seafood. These are called functional foods, because they have benefits beyond simply their nutrient content: calories, protein, fat, vitamins, and minerals. To do their magic, however, they must be part of a diet low in saturated fat, like the TLC diet, and they must be part of a dietary pattern, not just eaten as a single nutrient. Thus, it is crucial to eat a combination of these cholesterol-lowering foods in your everyday diet.

More than just your diet, however, is your mind-set and your motivation. That's why keeping a food journal is so important for kicking your program up a notch. Not only will it help you stay focused, it will also show you how to improve so you can make a change.

What If My Numbers Don't Drop?

Many people will be able to lower their LDL cholesterol with the TLC diet. This step-by-step plan allows you to lower your cholesterol by first reducing saturated fat, cholesterol, and trans fats; following a healthful diet; becoming physically active; reducing stress; and losing weight.

If after six weeks your blood cholesterol levels haven't changed or have changed very little, your doctor and/or health-care team will likely go over the principles of the TLC diet again, stressing the importance of adhering to the tenets of reducing saturated fat, trans fats, and cholesterol. If you are doing everything right and still nothing is working, your health-care team will likely add another dietary approach to your repertoire—they will encourage you to add more of these cholesterol-lowering, high-soluble fiber foods to your diet:

- *Plant stanols and sterols* (a type of plant fat)
- Beans and oatmeal
- Nuts and seeds
- Soy protein

DEFINITION

Plant stanols and sterols are naturally occurring fatlike compounds found in small amounts in whole grains, vegetables, fruits, nuts, seeds, and legumes. In the body, these plant compounds block cholesterol from being absorbed. I discuss plant stanols and sterols later in the chapter.

In a recent University of Toronto study, researchers looked at LDL levels of two groups of subjects. One was given a typical low-saturated-fat diet, and the other was given a low-saturated-fat diet with an emphasis on the four cholesterol-lowering foods just mentioned. After six months, both groups' LDL levels dropped, but the group with the cholesterol-lowering foods decreased LDL levels 14 percent more than the low-saturated-fat group. Improvements also appeared in the ratio of total cholesterol to HDL.

Increase Your Fiber

The typical TLC diet plan calls for about 20 to 30 grams of fiber per day, but on this more intense approach, you may want to up that even further. Current fiber dietary recommendations range from 21 to 38 grams depending on your age and calorie level, but clinical studies have shown people can eat more than that with no adverse effects.

Since soluble fiber is so important to lowering cholesterol, the TLC diet suggests getting 5 to 10 grams of soluble fiber a day and preferably 10 to 25 grams daily. But remember, no food contains 100 percent soluble fiber; food is a combination of both soluble and insoluble fiber.

Soluble fiber is found in a wide variety of foods but especially beans, certain whole grains like oats and barley, vegetables, and some fruits. The following table lists soluble fiber and total fiber amounts (in grams) for various foods:

	Soluble Fiber (in grams)	Total Fiber (in grams)
Whole-grain cereals		
Barley (1/2 cup cooked)	1	4
Oatbran (1/2 cup cooked)	1	3
Oatmeal (1/2 cup cooked)	1	2
Psyllium seeds, ground (1 TB.)	5	6
Fruit		
Apple (1 medium)	1	4
Banana (1 medium)	1	3
Blackberries (1/2 cup)	1	4
Citrus (orange, grapefruit; 1 medium)	2	2–3
Nectarine (1 medium)	1	2
Peach (1 medium)	1	2
Pear (1 medium)	2	4
Plum (1 medium)	1	1.5
Prunes (1/4 cup)	1.5	3
Legumes		
Black beans (1/2 cup cooked)	2	5.5
Black-eyed peas (1/2 cup cooked)	1	5.5
Chickpeas (1/2 cup cooked)	1	6
Kidney beans (1/2 cup cooked)	3	6
Lentils (1/2 cup cooked)	1	8
Lima beans (1/2 cup cooked)	3.5	6.5

continues

continued

	Soluble Fiber (in grams)	Total Fiber (in grams)
Navy beans (1/2 cup cooked)	2	6
Northern beans (1/2 cup cooked)	1.5	5.5
Pinto beans (1/2 cup cooked)	2	7
Vegetables		
Broccoli (1/2 cup cooked)	1	1.5
Brussels sprouts (1/2 cup cooked)	3	4.5
Carrots (1/2 cup cooked)	1	2.5

From Your Guide to Lowering Your Cholesterol With Therapeutic Lifestyle Changes, *courtesy of the National Heart, Lung, and Blood Institute.*

The key to success here is including a wide variety of foods that contain fiber, such as whole grains (rye, barley, oats, whole wheat, and so on), fruits, vegetables, and legumes.

The biggest problem with high-fiber diets occurs when people go from having a no-fiber or low-fiber diet to eating a high-fiber diet virtually overnight. Cramping, diarrhea, and gastrointestinal gas are some of the problems associated with a sudden increase in fiber. To minimize these results you should start slowly, gradually increasing your fiber intake over six to eight weeks.

You also need to remember to drink a lot of liquids to keep things flowing. If you do feel any discomfort, like gas or bloating, from upping your fiber intake, drop your level for a while and then try again, gradually increasing it. Remember, it may take your body a month or two to adjust to your new fiber intake, so give yourself a chance.

Most of your fiber should be in the form of soluble fiber. Also known as viscous fibers, these foods move through the system absorbing water and taking cholesterol with them, to be excreted later. In the Canadian study focusing on a diet pattern including cholesterol-lowering foods, viscous fibers alone reduced LDL cholesterol by 4 percent.

Soluble fibers are found in pectins, gums, mucilages, and some hemicelluloses, and they dissolve easily in water. Some foods high in soluble fibers are oats; oat bran; barley; rye; apples; oranges; pears; dried plums; grapefruits; lemons; limes; broccoli; carrots; legumes like beans, lentils, and chickpeas; and seeds. Let's look at some of the easier ones to add to your diet.

Home in on Oatmeal

Most people are familiar with oatmeal's potent cholesterol-lowering properties, and this link has only grown stronger in the last 10 years since the Food and Drug Administration approved an oatmeal health claim on labels. The claim states that "3 grams of soluble fiber daily from oatmeal, in a diet low in saturated fat and cholesterol, may reduce the risk of heart disease." This soluble oat fiber is a form of beta-glucan. Recent studies suggest that the fiber (beta-glucan) in oatmeal can do even more:

- Reduce the susceptibility of LDL to oxidation (stickiness)
- Reduce early hardening of the arteries
- Reduce the risk of high blood pressure, type 2 diabetes, and weight gain
- Aid in weight loss

If you're a breakfast eater and like oatmeal, I recommend a daily bowl of it at least five times a week. Since oatmeal can be dressed with so many different fruits, nuts, nut butters, and sweet spices, you're not likely to get bored (Chapter 15 has several oatmeal recipes). If you're not a fan of oatmeal for breakfast, there are other ways to get some of this nutritious high-fiber food:

- Put it (cooked or dry) in a smoothie, like an oatmeal shake.
- Use it in a side dish, such as Oatmeal Mushroom Ris-oatto (see Chapter 16).
- Bake it into cookies and muffins.
- Top it on fruit cobblers or crumbs.
- Mix it into breadcrumbs.
- Grind it into a flour and use it in place of some all-purpose flour.

Bring on the Beans

Beans are loaded with heart-protecting nutrients, including potassium, magnesium, folate, and fiber. In fact, 1 cup of cooked beans contains 4 grams of soluble fiber. One serving of beans equals about ½ cup, so all you need is four servings of beans a week—about 2 cups cooked—to lower your risk of heart disease by 22 percent.

Here are some ways to up your bean intake:

- Add beans to soup.
- Toss beans in green salads, pasta salads, and vegetable salads.
- Combine different types of beans to make colorful side dishes.
- Purée beans to make dips and spreads.
- Make bean burgers.
- Mix together beans and rice, and season with your favorite herbs.
- Experiment with black beans in brownies or chocolate cake.

Add a Little Flaxseed to Your Life

Like all high-fiber foods, flaxseed contains both soluble and insoluble fiber. It also has omega-3 fatty acids and a beneficial phytochemical called lignans. In addition to improving digestion and lowering cholesterol, flaxseed thins the blood, making it less sticky and reducing the risk of atherosclerotic plaque.

Whole flaxseed is better than flaxseed oil, but if you purchase whole flaxseed, be sure to grind it in a coffee or spice grinder first. Whole seeds will pass through your system undigested. All you need to reap the benefits of flaxseed is 1 to 2 tablespoons every few days. Here are some of my favorite ways to use it:

- Stir into oatmeal.
- Mix into yogurt.
- Put in smoothies.
- Add to muffins, bread, or pancake batter.
- Toss into a breadcrumb mixture for breading chicken, fish, or vegetables.

HEART-SMART HABITS

Keep flaxseed in the freezer. Freezing keeps the flaxseed from oxidizing and losing its nutritional potency. Flaxseed stored in whole form lasts longer than in ground form.

Increase Your Intake of Plant Foods

Eating a plant-based diet is the best thing you can do for your heart and your health. In addition to protecting you against heart disease, plant foods reduce your risk of cancer, diabetes, high blood pressure, obesity, and a host of other conditions. So what exactly is a plant-based diet? *Most* of your foods or a substantial amount should come from fruits, vegetables, beans, and whole grains, which should be minimally processed and in their fresh form. Contrary to popular belief, this doesn't mean that you have to go meat free and become a vegetarian. Animal and fish proteins and foods are simply not the center of the plate, but are a side or condiment, a small flavoring ingredient. Plan for several meatless meals a week, though.

Although plant foods contain dozens of beneficial phytochemicals and nutrients, when it comes to lowering your cholesterol, plant proteins like soy (which I talk about later in this chapter) and plant stanols and sterols are most important. Here's what you need to know about them.

Stanols and Sterols

Plant stanols and sterols are naturally occurring substances found in small amounts in many whole grains, fruits, vegetables, legumes, nuts, and seeds. They resemble cholesterol in structure and are sometimes called, as a group, phytosterols. In the body, stanols and sterols block absorption of cholesterol from the intestines, increasing excretion. Studies show that just 2 grams per day can lower LDL cholesterol by as much as 15 percent in weeks.

Getting that much, however, isn't as easy as it sounds. Naturally occurring sources like vegetable oils, salad dressings, milk, and nuts are high in calories and don't contain large amounts. For this reason, companies have begun fortifying foods like margarine, orange juice, and yogurt with these plant compounds. If you are taking a more intense dietary approach, including these foods in your diet is a good idea. But don't go overboard. While 2 grams can be helpful, eating 3 grams or more is not. That's because too much plant sterols and stanols can interfere with beta-carotene absorption and possibly other fat-soluble vitamins.

GOTCHA!

The American Heart Association recommends stanol- and sterol-fortified foods only for people who have high cholesterol levels or those who have already had a heart attack.

Vegetables and Fruits

Both vegetables and fruits are filled with antioxidants, anti-inflammatory agents and phytochemicals that shield the body from damaging free radicals and protect us from heart disease. The key is to eat enough.

Most people readily accept fruits, but if you eat too much, the calories can rack up fast. Vegetables, on the other hand, are lower in calories and often higher in fiber, but they lack the glamour and popularity of fruit.

Unfortunately, many people are turned off by what they perceive as bitter-tasting vegetables, and some people are more sensitive to bitter tastes than others. People who are more sensitive to bitter tastes are referred to as supertasters and tend to avoid vegetables. These are actually genetic differences and may explain why some people love broccoli while others hate it. If you are one of those picky eaters, it is still possible to enjoy vegetables. Consider the following ideas:

- Drizzle vegetables with olive oil and/or a sprinkle of nuts.
- Season your vegetables well with herbs and spices.
- Experiment with different cooking techniques. For instance, some people hate boiled brussels sprouts yet love roasted ones. The flavor is very different.
- Try adding a small spoonful of sugar or honey to stronger-tasting vegetables.
- Combine vegetables with other foods you like. For example, eat your mashed potatoes with peas and carrots.

What About Soy Protein?

Soy protein typically reduces cholesterol by around 2 percent. That's not a lot, but in combination with other cholesterol-lowering foods, it adds up. Plus, soy is a good replacement for saturated fat; products like tofu are good substitutes for fatty meat. In studies, soy has been shown to lower LDL and raise HDL cholesterol, but the effect has been small. Consequently, organizations like the American Heart Association have backed off on recommending soy protein other than as a replacement for saturated fat. However, the jury is still out regarding this issue, as studies showing the benefit of soy on heart disease continue to roll in.

Nevertheless, the Food and Drug Administration does allow manufacturers with soy products containing 6.25 grams of soy protein per serving to state that diets that include 25 grams of soy protein daily and are low in saturated fat and cholesterol may reduce the risk of heart disease.

Recently, soy protein has also been found to benefit blood pressure by lowering systolic (the top number) blood pressure.

The advantages of soy come from food, not supplements. Nutritionally, they are low in saturated fat; have no cholesterol; and contain polyunsaturated fats, fiber, vitamins, and minerals, making them well worth adding to your diet. Here are a few ways to add more soy to your life:

- Drink soy milk.
- Make tofu a main entrée.
- Try soy burgers, sausages, and soy meats.
- Munch on some soy nuts.
- Add edamame to soups and salads.
- Experiment with other soy products, like tempeh.

Go for Nuts and Seeds

Nuts and seeds are nutritional powerhouses loaded with good-for-you vitamins and minerals. In addition to lowering cholesterol, nuts may improve dilation of blood vessels, reduce inflammation, combat blood pressure, moderate blood sugar levels, and aid in weight loss.

Adding nuts and seeds to your diet is easy as long as you think of them as a food, not simply an add-on. Use nuts in place of fatty, salty snacks like chips. Toss them with vegetables and in a stir-fry, sprinkle on top of salads in place of cheese, use them ground in sauces (nut butters are good for this), or add them to fresh fruit or nonfat yogurt for dessert.

GOTCHA!

Nuts are easy to overeat, and calories rack up fast. Don't grab handfuls of nuts out of a can or eat them mindlessly. Instead, portion out the amount you want and then put away the jar or can.

Kick It Up a Notch with Seafood

Fatty fish is an excellent source of omega-3 fatty acids. Although omega-3 fatty acids don't lower LDL, they provide plenty of other heart-healthy advantages, like preventing blood clots, reducing inflammation, and keeping your heart rhythm working smoothly. This makes them a good choice on this list and part of your diet several times a week.

Many people shy away from eating fish because they don't know how to cook it, but preparing fish is easier than you think. Start slow, either broiling or sautéing your fish. Then you can dress it up with sauces and side dishes. If you're still not sure of what to do, check out cookbooks, blogs, food TV shows, and YouTube videos. A lot of high-quality seafood is available in cans or, more recently, pouches. Some of my favorites are sardines, salmon, and tuna. And don't be afraid to experiment—my Sicilian Sardine Pasta (see Chapter 19) is to die for!

The TLC diet is a powerful tool for lowering cholesterol and improving your health, but sometimes it may not be enough. If that's the case and your doctor does prescribe cholesterol-lowering medication, don't be disheartened—and don't give up on your TLC diet. By sticking to your TLC diet, you'll be able to take the lowest dose of medication, not to mention all the other health benefits you will be receiving, like more energy, better weight management, and reduced risk of diabetes and stroke.

Keep a Food Journal

Keeping a food journal is another tool for helping you achieve the benefits of the TLC diet and enjoy good health. In a food journal, you write down everything you eat and drink in one day. It is also a good idea to include physical activity in this list.

You can do this with an old-fashioned pen and paper, or you can use an online journal. Online journals can be accessed through your smartphone (there are now apps for this), iPod, or computer, and includes sites like myfooddiary.com, fitday.com, and sparkpeople.com, to name a few.

The purpose of a food journal is to see how close you've come to adhering to the TLC diet pattern and to track your progress. You can do this in two ways. First, you can tally up calories, saturated fat, cholesterol, and sodium, and see if these numbers fit with your plan (see Chapter 2 for specifics). This is easy to do if you use an online program, which usually automatically calculates numbers. Second, you can do this by looking at food groups and seeing if your diet fits the TLC pattern (such as 8 to 10 servings of fruits and vegetables a day, 5 ounces or less of lean protein, 2 to 3 servings of nonfat dairy, and 5 or 6 servings of whole grains, depending on your calorie level). Here you need to pay particular attention to serving sizes.

There are other benefits, too. The simple act of writing down what you eat encourages you to eat less and eat better, by increasing your awareness of what, how much, and why you're eating. It can identify the type of eater you are (for example, a grazer versus someone who eats just three meals a day) and your typical eating patterns so you can adjust those accordingly. It can reveal triggers to avoid, such as overeating when eating out or drinking too many calories.

HEART-SMART HABITS

People who keep detailed food journals lose more weight and keep the weight off better than people who don't journal. One large study tracking 1,700 people found that people who kept a journal lost twice as much weight as those who kept no records.

What to Include

How much information you want to put in your food journal depends on you, but basically, more is better. Here's what you should include to start:

Date

What you ate (for example: sandwich includes bread, cheese, turkey, and mustard)

How much you ate (specific portion sizes, like $\frac{1}{2}$ cup oatmeal or 1 cup vanilla yogurt)

Preparation method (baked, broiled, and so on)

What time you ate it

Where you were (at the table, watching TV, and so on)

Who you were with (family, friend(s), or alone)

Exercise you did that day

Mood you were in

Tips for Successful Journaling

Keep your journal with you wherever you go, and write down what you ate as soon as you finish eating it. If you wait, you will likely forget some things. Also do this with exercise. Here are some other tips:

- Write down *everything* you eat and drink, including candy, snacks, tastes, bites, and water. This can add up quickly. Americans typically underestimate their food intake by 20 to 40 percent.
- Be as detailed and accurate as possible. This means measuring and weighing all your food, at least at first, so you can keep track of portion sizes. As time goes on, you'll get better at eyeballing amounts.
- Review your journal weekly. Consult with a health professional, if possible, and make changes accordingly. A dietitian can help you evaluate your food journal and give you suggestions on how to improve or change your diet.
- Be vigilant—remember, your health is worth it!

The Least You Need to Know

- If your cholesterol levels aren't dropping, consider upping your intake of cholesterol-lowering foods high in soluble fiber like oatmeal, beans, barley, plant stanols, and nuts.
- Although soy protein doesn't lower cholesterol as much as once thought, it is a good replacement for foods high in saturated fat and should be included on the TLC diet.
- People with high cholesterol and/or heart disease should include more plant stanols and sterols in their diet, in the form of whole plant foods and fortified foods like margarine.
- Eating seafood high in omega-3 fatty acids like salmon, tuna, mackerel, and sardines has many heart-healthy benefits.
- Keep a food journal to track your progress and setbacks and help develop strategies and techniques for achieving a healthful TLC lifestyle.

Part 4

Cooking the TLC Way

With a pantry and refrigerator full of healthful food and a bunch of menus to match, there's only one thing left to do: get cooking. Preparing and serving healthful food for you and your family is more than just the right thing to do. It shows your family members that you love them and proves that healthful food can be fast, delicious, and satisfying. This part of the book has 80 recipes, and each one is low in saturated fat and cholesterol. But this is no "diet food." Each meal is high in taste and flavor. Since plant food is so important, a whole chapter is devoted to vegetarian and vegan options. There's also a chapter dedicated to beans and grains, another important component of the TLC diet. I've included a chapter of on-the-run meals for when you don't have time to cook but still want to eat something healthful. Finally, don't forget to save room for the desserts in the last chapter!

Chapter

15

Breaking Fast

In This Chapter

- Let's hear it for oats!
- Perfect pancakes and muffins
- Super smoothies and shakes
- Extra-special eggs

Traditional American breakfasts leave much to be desired when it comes to heart health. Bacon, eggs, and sausage; pancakes drenched in butter and syrup; and sugary cereal are typically low in fiber and high in calories, fat, saturated fat, cholesterol, and/or sugar—not the best choices on the TLC diet. In this chapter, I give ideas on how to lighten up your morning meal and start your day with healthful, nutritious, and delicious foods that will rev up your engine, keep your heart running smoothly, and provide you with plenty of eye-opening energy.

I start with an old-fashioned favorite: oatmeal. Oatmeal is high in soluble fiber, fills you up, and is inexpensive. It's also versatile and can be sweet or savory, depending on how you like it (check out the Oatmeal Mushroom Ris-oatto in Chapter 16). Most of the oatmeal recipes in this chapter are on the sweet side but will still have you thinking of oatmeal in a new way, like the Banana Oatmeal Peanut Butter Shake.

Next, I move on to pancakes, bread, and muffins. These are great make-ahead breakfasts—yes, even the pancakes—you can reheat and eat the next day. I like to individually wrap muffins and bread (in pieces) and freeze right away. Pull them out the night before or even in the morning, and by the time you get to the office, they're defrosted and ready to eat.

Smoothies are another quick and filling breakfast that you can whip up in a matter of minutes, as long as you have the right ingredients. The beauty of smoothies is that almost anything and particularly any fruit can be the right ingredient! My favorite Sunshine Orange Smoothie tastes like you're drinking an orange.

Finally, I offer up some egg dishes. Made with egg whites and chock-full of vegetables, these are filling, low-calorie breakfasts—and you won't even miss the yolks. Wrap them up in a whole-wheat tortilla for quick meal on the run, or pair them with fruit and hot tea or coffee, and you've got yourself a morning meal fit for a king or queen!

Nutty Chocolate Cherry Almond Bars

Almond butter and honey keep these dense bars—chock-full of high-fiber nuts, seeds, and oatmeal—together. Don't be fooled by their small size. Paired with a glass of milk and a piece of fruit, they make a filling and satisfying meal.

Yield:	**Prep time:**	**Cook time:**	**Serving size:**
15 bars	15 minutes	5 minutes plus time to chill in refrigerator (1 hour or overnight)	1 bar
Each serving has:			
217 calories	12 g fat	1 g saturated fat	0 mg cholesterol
3 g fiber	4 mg sodium		

1 cup regular old-fashioned oats

1 cup puffed kamut, wheat, or rice cereal

1/4 cup ground flaxseeds

2 TB. sesame seeds

2 TB. poppy seeds

1 TB. sunflower seeds

1/2 cup chopped almonds

1/3 cup chopped dried figs

1/3 cup chopped dried cherries

3/4 cup almond butter

1 tsp. vanilla extract

1/2 cup honey

3 TB. turbinado sugar

2 TB. unsweetened cocoa powder

1. Line an 8×8 or 9×9 baking pan with a piece of foil, leaving a 1-inch overhang on each long side. Spray with cooking spray.
2. Toast old-fashioned oats in medium pan over medium-high heat, stirring constantly until they turn slightly brown and begin to smell nutty. Set aside.
3. In a large bowl, mix puffed kamut, flaxseeds, sesame seeds, poppy seeds, sunflower seeds, almonds, figs, cherries, and cooled oatmeal.
4. Combine almond butter, vanilla extract, honey, turbinado sugar, and unsweetened cocoa powder in a small saucepan and stir over low heat until blended and smooth, about 5 minutes.

5. Pour almond butter mixture into oat mixture and mix until dry ingredients are moistened. Transfer mixture to the baking pan, and press with a piece of plastic wrap firmly and evenly to make a layer. Cover and refrigerate at least 1 hour or overnight.
6. When cold, use the foil to remove from the pan and transfer to the cutting board. Cut into 15 bars.

GOTCHA!

Honey and maple syrup may seem like more healthful sweeteners, but in the body, they act just like any other concentrated sugar. Use them sparingly, and you'll do just fine.

Cranberry Nut Muesli

Dried cranberries, almonds, peanuts, and oats give this *muesli* its characteristic taste. Toast the oats in a dry pan for a more nutty flavor. Eat it plain or mixed with milk or yogurt.

Yield:	**Prep time:**	**Serving size:**
$2\frac{1}{2}$ cups	5 minutes	$\frac{1}{4}$ cup
Each serving has:		
166 calories	10 g fat	2 g saturated fat
0 mg cholesterol	3 g fiber	24 mg sodium

1 cup regular old-fashioned oats
$\frac{1}{2}$ cup peanuts, salted
$\frac{1}{2}$ cup almonds, whole or chopped
4 TB. mini chocolate chips
4 TB. dried cranberries
2 TB. unsalted pumpkin seeds
Pinch salt (optional)

1. Mix together old-fashioned oats, peanuts, almonds, chocolate chips, cranberries, pumpkin seeds, and salt (if using) in a medium bowl.
2. Store in an airtight container (will keep at room temperature).

Variation: For **Apple Cranberry Muesli,** mix $\frac{1}{4}$ cranberry muesli with $\frac{1}{2}$ apple, cored, peeled, and shredded; $\frac{1}{8}$ teaspoon lemon juice; $\frac{1}{8}$ teaspoon cinnamon; and $\frac{1}{2}$ cup nonfat milk or unsweetened soy milk. Serve immediately. Makes one individual portion.

DEFINITION

Muesli is a dry, uncooked cereal composed of rolled oats, nuts, and fruits. It was introduced by a Swiss physician in the early twentieth century and inspired by shepherds in the Alps who ate oats, raisins, apples, and nuts for breakfast.

Overnight Pineapple Coconut Oatmeal

Sweet pineapple and coconut give oatmeal a tropical flavor. Letting it sit overnight softens the oatmeal so it's chewy but ready to heat and eat in seconds. Top with sliced banana, almonds, and flaxseeds for some extra fiber and crunch.

Yield:	**Prep time:**	**Cook time:**	**Serving size:**
$1\frac{1}{2}$ cups	5 minutes	1 minute	$\frac{3}{4}$ cup
Each serving has:			
316 calories	9 g fat	2 g saturated fat	0 mg cholesterol
8 g fiber	84 mg sodium		

1 cup regular old-fashioned oats
1 cup nonfat milk or almond milk
3 TB. crushed or chopped pineapple
$\frac{1}{2}$ tsp. honey
1 TB. sweetened coconut
10 whole almonds, chopped
Dash nutmeg
1 banana, sliced
1 TB. ground flaxseeds

1. In a medium bowl, mix old-fashioned oats, nonfat milk, pineapple, honey, coconut, almonds, and nutmeg. Cover and place in the refrigerator overnight.
2. The next morning, heat oatmeal in the microwave for 40 seconds or until warm. Add sliced banana and stir in flaxseeds. Serve immediately.

Variation: You can use any combination of fruit and nuts for overnight oatmeal. Other favorite flavors include maple syrup (in place of the honey), walnuts, and raisins; or pecans, apples, and cinnamon.

GOTCHA!

Coconut meat is better than coconut oil or coconut milk, but 1 tablespoon shredded coconut still contains nearly 2 grams of saturated fat, along with some fiber, potassium, and magnesium. Use it sparingly.

Teff Oatmeal with Blueberries

Although you can use any fresh fruit in this hearty hot cereal blend, I like the taste of the sweet-tart blueberries. If you want more crunch and sweetness, serve it with sliced bananas or pears and chopped or sliced almonds.

Yield:	**Prep time:**	**Cook time:**	**Serving size:**
$2\frac{1}{2}$ cups	10 minutes	20 minutes	$\frac{1}{2}$ cup
Each serving has:			
129 calories	3 g fat	.3 g saturated fat	0 mg cholesterol
3 g fiber	10 mg sodium		

$\frac{1}{4}$ cup whole-grain *teff*

$1\frac{3}{4}$ cups water

$\frac{1}{2}$ cup old-fashioned oats

1 TB. ground flaxseeds

1 cup blueberries

1 TB. almond butter

1 TB. honey

$\frac{1}{4}$ tsp. cinnamon

$\frac{1}{4}$ cup nonfat plain Greek-style yogurt

1. Toast whole-grain teff in a medium saucepan over medium-high heat, stirring constantly for about 1 to 2 minutes. Teff will begin to smell nutty.
2. Add water, bring to boil, and cook 10 minutes. Mix in old-fashioned oats, bring back to a boil, and simmer for 5 more minutes or until oatmeal is done.
3. Take oatmeal-teff mixture off heat and stir in flaxseeds, blueberries, almond butter, honey, and cinnamon. Mix in nonfat Greek-style yogurt right before serving.

DEFINITION

Originating in Ethiopia, **teff** is a tiny brown grain that cooks up creamy and has a pungent, nutty taste. It's most known as the main ingredient in injera, a spongy Ethiopian bread.

Multigrain Pancakes with Maple Peaches

Buckwheat flour and spelt flour give these multigrain pancakes their edge, and peaches flavored with maple syrup are the topping.

Yield:	**Prep time:**	**Cook time:**	**Serving size:**
12 3½-inch pancakes and 2 cups peaches	10 minutes	10 minutes	3 pancakes and ½ cup peaches
Each serving has:			
231 calories	4 g fat	.6 g saturated fat	53 mg cholesterol
5 g fiber	262 mg sodium		

3 large peaches, peeled, pitted, and diced (about 2 cups)

2 tsp. vanilla extract

2 TB. maple syrup

½ cup *white whole-wheat flour*

¼ cup spelt flour

¼ cup buckwheat flour

1 tsp. baking powder

¼ tsp. baking soda

2 tsp. granulated sugar

Pinch salt

1 tsp. corn or canola oil

1 egg (or 2 TB. egg substitute)

1¼ cups buttermilk

1 tsp. orange juice

1. In a medium bowl, mix peaches, 1 teaspoon vanilla extract, and maple syrup. Set aside.
2. Heat an electric griddle to 350°F, or place a griddle pan over medium-high heat. Spray with cooking spray. In a large bowl, mix white whole-wheat flour, spelt flour, buckwheat flour, baking powder, baking soda, sugar, and salt.
3. In another bowl, blend corn oil, egg, buttermilk, orange juice, and remaining 1 teaspoon vanilla.
4. Pour liquid ingredients into dry ingredients and gently mix just until incorporated. Let sit for 5 minutes. Mixture will get thicker.
5. Place about 2 tablespoons batter per pancake onto the prepared griddle and cook about 2 minutes, then flip and cook for another 2 minutes.

6. To serve, place $\frac{1}{2}$ cup peach mixture on top of 3 multigrain pancakes.

DEFINITION

White whole-wheat flour is a whole-wheat flour, meaning it contains both the bran and the germ. It is made from a different type of wheat (white wheat) that is lighter in color and milder in taste than typical whole-wheat flour, which is made from red wheat.

Whole-Wheat Banana Bread Pancakes with Walnuts

These light, airy banana pancakes are so good they don't even need syrup. They're flavored with cinnamon and vanilla and a touch of sugar—just add some fresh fruit for a sweet yet satisfying breakfast.

Yield:	**Prep time:**	**Cook time:**	**Serving size:**
10 3-inch pancakes	10 minutes	10 minutes	5 pancakes
Each serving has:			
450 calories	14 g fat	1 g saturated fat	0 mg cholesterol
10 g fiber	507 mg sodium		

1 cup white whole-wheat flour
1½ tsp. baking powder
⅛ tsp. kosher salt
1 egg white (or 4 TB. egg substitute)
2 medium bananas, mashed
½ tsp. cinnamon
1 tsp. vanilla extract
1 TB. plus 1 tsp. corn oil
2 tsp. granulated sugar
1 TB. plus 1 tsp. chopped walnuts

1. In a medium bowl, mix white whole-wheat flour, baking powder, kosher salt, egg white, bananas, cinnamon, vanilla extract, corn oil, sugar, and walnuts until incorporated. Do not overmix.
2. Heat an electric griddle to 350°F, or place a griddle pan over medium-high heat. Spray with cooking spray. Spoon 3-inch pancakes onto the hot pan. Cook for about 2 minutes, then flip. Pancakes will be brown on the bottom and you will begin to see bubbles forming on top. Flip and cook 2 minutes more, checking so pancakes don't get too brown.
3. Serve immediately with fresh fruit like strawberries or blueberries.

Variation: These pancakes use bananas, but other fruit (or vegetables) also work. Consider experimenting with pumpkin purée, wild blueberries, or apples. You can also vary the flours with oatmeal, almond, spelt, or buckwheat flour.

Pumpkin Ginger Bread

Candied ginger gives this moist pumpkin bread some spice, while flaxseed adds substance, making it a good choice for breakfast or a snack.

Yield:	**Prep time:**	**Cook time:**	**Serving size:**
12 pieces ($2\frac{1}{4}$ by $2\frac{3}{4}$ inches each)	15 minutes	25 to 30 minutes	1 piece
Each serving has:			
125 calories	2 g fat	0 g saturated fat	18 mg cholesterol
2 g fiber	240 mg sodium		

1 cup white whole-wheat flour
$\frac{1}{2}$ cup all-purpose flour
$\frac{1}{4}$ cup ground flaxseeds
$\frac{1}{2}$ tsp. sea salt
1 tsp. baking soda
$\frac{1}{2}$ tsp. baking powder
$\frac{1}{2}$ cup brown sugar
$\frac{1}{2}$ cup unsweetened applesauce
1 cup pumpkin purée
$\frac{1}{3}$ cup corn or canola oil
1 egg
2 egg whites
$\frac{1}{3}$ cup nonfat plain Greek-style yogurt
$1\frac{1}{2}$ tsp. pumpkin pie spice
2 TB. chopped candied ginger

1. Preheat the oven to 350°F. Spray a 9×9 square baking pan with cooking spray. In a medium bowl, mix white whole-wheat flour, all-purpose flour, flaxseeds, sea salt, baking soda, and baking powder.
2. In a separate bowl, mix brown sugar, unsweetened applesauce, pumpkin purée, corn oil, egg, egg whites, nonfat Greek-style yogurt, and pumpkin pie spice. Pour liquid ingredients into dry ingredients and mix until just incorporated. Do not overmix. Fold in candied ginger.
3. Pour batter into the prepared pan, and bake in the oven 25 to 30 minutes or until a toothpick inserted comes out clean and cake pulls away from pan. Cut into 12 pieces.
4. For best results, store in the refrigerator. Keeps for 3 to 5 days.

HEALTHFUL LIVING

Pumpkin is a highly nutritious vegetable. Cooked similarly to squash, it is loaded with beta-carotene (the plant form of vitamin A), zeaxanthine (which is good for the eyes), and a slew of B vitamins.

Morning Glory Muffins

With apples, raisins, pineapple, and carrots, these moist little gems are chock-full of high-fiber fruits and vegetables. Keep them in the freezer for a go-to snack or breakfast when you don't have time to prepare something.

Yield: 16 muffins	**Prep time:** 5 minutes	**Cook time:** 16 minutes	**Serving size:** 1 muffin
Each serving has:			
176 calories	7 g fat	1 g saturated fat	0 mg cholesterol
2 g fiber	219 mg sodium		

1 cup all-purpose flour

1 cup white whole-wheat flour

$\frac{1}{2}$ cup brown sugar, lightly packed

2 tsp. baking soda

2 tsp. cinnamon

$\frac{1}{4}$ tsp. salt

$\frac{1}{4}$ cup egg substitute or 1 large egg

$\frac{1}{2}$ cup vegetable oil

$\frac{1}{2}$ cup unsweetened applesauce

$\frac{1}{2}$ cup crushed pineapple

$\frac{1}{4}$ cup shredded sweetened coconut

1 tsp. vanilla extract

1 cup small chopped apple, unpeeled (the smaller, the better)

$\frac{1}{3}$ cup raisins

$\frac{3}{4}$ cup grated carrots

1. Preheat the oven to 350°F. Line a muffin pan with paper or foil liners or spray with cooking spray.
2. In a bowl, combine all-purpose flour, white whole-wheat flour, brown sugar, baking soda, cinnamon, and salt. Whisk to blend evenly.
3. In a separate bowl, whisk together egg substitute, vegetable oil, unsweetened applesauce, pineapple, sweetened coconut, and vanilla extract. Stir in apple, raisins, and carrots. Add to flour mixture and blend just until moistened but still lumpy.
4. Spoon batter into muffin cups, filling each cup about two thirds full. Bake until springy to the touch, about 16 minutes.
5. Let cool for 5 minutes, then transfer to a wire rack and let cool completely. Tightly sealed in a cool place, muffins will keep for several days.

HEART-SMART HABITS

Not only is using applesauce a good way to add sweetness with less sugar, but it can also replace some of the fat, like butter or oil, in muffin or bread recipes like banana or zucchini bread. The applesauce keeps bread moist without the extra fat.

Banana Oatmeal Peanut Butter Shake

Cooked oatmeal is the secret ingredient in this high-fiber, nutritious, and filling shake loaded with peanut butter, flaxseed, and soy milk.

Yield:	**Prep time:**	**Cook time:**	**Serving size:**
24 ounces	5 minutes	5 minutes	12 ounces
Each serving has:			
248 calories	7 g fat	1 g saturated fat	0 mg cholesterol
6 g fiber	62 mg sodium		

1 cup water

½ cup old-fashioned oats

1 TB. all-natural unsalted peanut butter

1 TB. ground flaxseeds

1 cup ice cubes

1 cup soy milk

1 tsp. honey

1 banana

Pinch cinnamon

1. Heat water in a small saucepot until boiling. Add old-fashioned oats, reduce heat, and cook about 5 minutes until done. Set aside and let cool for about 10 minutes.
2. Place cooled oatmeal, peanut butter, flaxseeds, ice cubes, soy milk, honey, banana, and cinnamon in a blender. Purée for about 2 minutes until smooth.
3. Divide into two glasses and serve immediately.

Variation: For a frosty drink, freeze the banana for about an hour before blending.

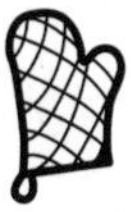

HEART-SMART HABITS

As the oatmeal sits, it absorbs liquid. Thus, if you want to save this drink for the next day, you'll probably have to add 6 to 8 ounces more milk to it.

Super Strawberry Carrot Smoothie

Buy strawberries in peak season for this sweet smoothie. Carrot bumps up fiber as well as vitamins and minerals and mellows out the flavor while still whipping up as smooth as silk.

Yield: 2 cups	**Prep time:** 5 minutes	**Serving size:** 1 cup
Each serving has:		
65 calories	0 g fat	0 g saturated fat
0 mg cholesterol	4 g fiber	36 mg sodium

$1\frac{1}{2}$ cups sliced strawberries

1 carrot, peeled and cut into 1-in. pieces (about 3 oz.)

1 TB. honey

$\frac{1}{4}$ cup water

4 ice cubes

1. In a blender, place strawberries, carrot, honey, water, and ice cubes. Purée for about 1 minute until well blended.
2. Pour into two tall glasses and serve immediately.

HEART-SMART HABITS

Eat carrots for your eyes. One large carrot contains more than 240 percent of the recommended daily allowance for vitamin A (in the form of beta-carotene). Vitamin A protects eyes from damaging free radicals and slows the development of age-related macular degeneration.

Black and Blue Vanilla Smoothie

Blackberries and blueberries provide natural sweetness in this thick, creamy smoothie, pumped up with vanilla yogurt and vanilla soy milk.

Yield:	**Prep time:**	**Serving size:**
3 cups	5 minutes	1 cup
Each serving has:		
95 calories	0 g fat	0 g saturated fat
0 mg cholesterol	4 g fiber	48 mg sodium

- 1 cup blueberries
- 1 cup blackberries
- $\frac{1}{2}$ cup nonfat vanilla Greek-style yogurt
- 1 cup vanilla light soy milk
- $\frac{1}{2}$ cup ice cubes

1. Place blueberries, blackberries, nonfat vanilla Greek-style yogurt, vanilla soy milk, and ice cubes in a blender and purée on high for $1\frac{1}{2}$ to 2 minutes.
2. Pour into three tall glasses and serve immediately.

Variation: For an icy-cold smoothie, freeze berries before proceeding with recipe.

HEART-SMART HABITS

Berries are loaded with disease-fighting antioxidants, making them one of the superfruits you should have every day. Berry antioxidants help unclog arteries, protect cells from damage, and boost brain function.

Sunshine Orange Smoothie

This citrus smoothie tastes like a glass of sunshine. Since you use the whole orange, including the membranes, it's also high in fiber. Serve it at breakfast or anytime.

Yield:	**Prep time:**	**Serving size:**
4 cups	5 minutes	1 cup
Each serving has:		
88 calories	0 g fat	0 g saturated fat
0 mg cholesterol	3 g fiber	23 mg sodium

- 4 fresh seedless oranges, peeled (use different varieties for more flavor)
- 1 tsp. orange zest
- 2 cups ice cubes
- ½ cup plain unsweetened almond milk
- 1 tsp. vanilla
- 1 TB. honey

1. Place oranges, orange zest, ice cubes, unsweetened almond milk, and honey in a blender and purée for 1 minute until smooth.
2. Pour into four tall glasses and serve immediately.

HEALTHFUL LIVING

One large orange contains more than 150 percent of the recommended daily allowance for vitamin C. Vitamin C is an antioxidant that is involved in the growth and repair of cells (helps heal scars) and boosts iron and calcium absorption.

Tomato-Egg Scramble

Don't substitute ground cumin for cumin seed in this Indian-inspired recipe. The seed has a more intense flavor and crunch, which contrasts the creamy eggs and mild tomato. Fresh cilantro adds color as well as a burst of freshness.

Yield:	**Prep time:**	**Cook time:**	**Serving size:**
1½ cups	10 minutes	5 minutes	¾ cup
Each serving has:			
81 calories	3 g fat	0 g saturated fat	0 mg cholesterol
1 g fiber	119 mg sodium		

4 egg whites (or 1 cup egg substitute)

1 tsp. corn oil

1 clove garlic, minced

1 tsp. cumin seeds

½ small onion, finely chopped

½ medium tomato, seeded and chopped into ½-in. pieces

1 TB. finely chopped cilantro

Nonfat yogurt for garnish

1. Beat egg whites in a small bowl and set aside. Heat corn oil in a small pan over medium-high heat; when hot, add garlic and cumin seeds. Sauté, stirring frequently until fragrant and toasted, about 1 to 2 minutes. Add onion and cook for about 2 to 3 minutes or until onions are slightly brown and caramelized.
2. Pour in tomato and beaten egg whites. Let sit for 30 seconds before turning over with a spatula. Let cook another 30 seconds. Turn over again until egg whites are done, about 2 minutes. Top with cilantro and serve with a dollop of nonfat yogurt.

Variation: If you don't plan on having any other high-cholesterol foods the rest of the day, you can substitute 1 whole egg for 1 of the egg whites (1 whole egg plus ¾ cup egg whites).

HEALTHFUL LIVING

According to 2010 USDA data, eggs have 14 percent less cholesterol than they did 10 years ago, dropping from 215 mg cholesterol to 185 mg cholesterol. A change in the hen's diet, the way the animals are bred, and other factors may be the reasons for the decrease.

Spinach-Egg-Potato Scramble

Cooking the potatoes first reduces the cooking time and allows you to use less oil while still getting a velvety texture inside and a crisp outside. Combined with spinach, onions, and eggs, this makes a nice breakfast or light lunch.

Yield: 3 cups	**Prep time:** 10 minutes	**Cook time:** 20 minutes	**Serving size:** 1½ cups
Each serving has:			
124 calories	3 g fat	0 g saturated fat	0 mg cholesterol
3 g fiber	258 mg sodium		

2 small potatoes, unpeeled, diced into ¼-in. pieces (6 oz. total)

1 tsp. canola or corn oil

2 TB. finely chopped red onion

4 cups packed raw spinach

Pinch ground black pepper

⅛ tsp. sea salt (optional)

4 beaten egg whites (or 1 cup egg substitute)

1 tsp. any fresh chopped herbs (I like basil or oregano)

1. Fill a small pot with water and heat over medium-high heat until it boils. Add diced potatoes and lower heat until boiling slowly. Boil potatoes for about 6 minutes or until soft but still slightly firm. Drain, rinse with cold water to stop cooking, and set aside.
2. Heat a large skillet over medium-high heat. Add canola oil and cooled potatoes. Cook about 2 minutes on each side until potatoes begin to brown. Add red onion and spinach. Cook for another minute until onions begin to brown and spinach softens. Sprinkle with black pepper and sea salt (if using), then pour in beaten egg whites and chopped herbs. Scramble slightly, let set, and then flip in batches until cooked through, about 1 or 2 minutes. Serve immediately.

Variation: For **Spinach-Egg-Potato Sandwich,** wrap 1 serving of Spinach-Potato-Egg Scramble in an 8-inch whole-wheat tortilla with 2 slices of tomato and ½ tablespoon low-fat canola mayonnaise.

GOTCHA!

Read the label when buying egg substitutes. Some have fillers, emulsifiers, and coloring agents in them that affect quality and nutrition. This is also the reason amounts vary—for instance, for egg substitutes, 1 cup equals 4 egg whites, while in another, $\frac{3}{4}$ cup equals 4 egg whites. Try to buy only pure egg whites whenever possible, with no additives, fillers, or salt.

Chapter 16

Beans and Grains

In This Chapter

- Whole-grain pilafs and risottos
- Ideas for building up your bean repertoire
- Surprising burgers, burritos, and tacos

When it comes to lowering cholesterol, high-fiber foods are so vital to your success and good health that I've devoted an entire chapter to these foods. Upping your fiber intake—particularly your soluble fiber intake—can effectively lower your LDL cholesterol by 3 to 5 percent or more. These foods can also help you in other ways: by improving digestion, keeping you regular, supplying other beneficial nutrients, and filling you up with fewer calories. This last advantage is especially helpful if you're trying to lose weight and keep it off.

Although fiber is found in all kinds of fruits and vegetables, in this chapter, I focus on the two best sources: beans and whole grains. These are also the two food groups most Americans don't eat nearly enough of.

In this chapter, I show you some unusual and interesting ways to use whole grains, like in my Oatmeal Mushroom Ris-oatto; share a few tips on how to sneak more beans into your diet; and give you some options for creating your own high-fiber dishes.

With a few exceptions, most of these recipes supply between 4 and 10 grams of fiber per serving. Many of them also include a fiber boost, which is a food or foods you can add to up your fiber intake just a few more grams.

Think of these recipes as guidelines to help you develop your own unique bean and whole-grain meals. Don't like barley? Stick to brown rice or try quinoa or wild rice. Kidney beans aren't your favorite? Use black beans or pinto beans. The purpose of this chapter is to get you thinking about including some kind of bean or whole grain in nearly every meal—or at least four or five meals a week. If you do that, you'll be well on your way to a healthy heart and a healthy body.

Barley with Cherries, Pecans, and Honeyed Salmon

Fresh cherries and nutty pecans are tossed with orange-scented barley, then paired with baked salmon brushed with sweet-spicy honey. If fresh cherries aren't available, just use frozen instead.

Yield:	**Prep time:**	**Cook time:**	**Serving size:**
12 ounces salmon with 2 cups barley	10 minutes	1 hour	3 ounces salmon with ½ cup barley
Each serving has:			
308 calories	10 g fat	2 g saturated fat	47 mg cholesterol
6 g fiber	109 mg sodium		

½ cup hulled barley

1½ cups water

2 tsp. honey

¼ tsp. chili powder

1 tsp. low-sodium soy sauce

¼ tsp. ground ginger

4 (3-oz.) boneless, skinless salmon fillets

1 tsp. olive oil

¼ cup pecans, chopped

½ cup chopped fresh cherries or thawed frozen cherries

Juice of ½ orange (about 3 TB.)

1 tsp. orange zest

½ cup loosely packed Italian parsley, chopped

Pinch freshly ground black pepper

1. Cook barley in water in 1½-quart pot according to package directions. Set aside. This can be done a day ahead of time.
2. Preheat the oven to 450°F. In a small bowl, mix honey, chili powder, low-sodium soy sauce, and ginger. Rub on salmon fillets and place on a plate. Set aside and let marinate for 15 minutes.
3. Heat olive oil in a small nonstick sauté pan over medium-high heat until hot. Add pecans, stirring constantly for about 20 seconds, until nuts smell toasted. Set aside.
4. In a large bowl, mix hot cooked barley with pecans, fresh cherries, orange juice, orange zest, Italian parsley, and black pepper. Set aside.

5. Spray a baking sheet with cooking spray. Place salmon fillets on the prepared baking sheet and bake in the oven for about 5 minutes or until done (when fish flakes easily).
6. To serve, place $\frac{1}{2}$ cup barley mixture on each of four plates and top with 1 salmon fillet.

Fiber Boost: Add $\frac{1}{4}$ cup steamed chopped kale to 1 serving of barley mixture before topping with salmon.

HEALTHFUL LIVING

Unlike other grains, fiber is found throughout the barley kernel, not just in the bran. Hulled and hull-less barley are the least processed and most nutritious kinds on the market. You can also find pearled barley (polished barley) and quick-cooking barley, which is pearled barley that has been rolled and thinly shaved so it cooks a bit more quickly. Both hulled and pearled barley take a little less than an hour to cook.

Oatmeal Mushroom Ris-oatto

You'll be surprised at how creamy and cheesy this healthful version of a *risotto* made with oatmeal tastes. Flecked with green peas, it makes a filling, nutritious, and colorful entrée or hearty side.

Yield:	**Prep time:**	**Cook time:**	**Serving size:**
$2\frac{1}{2}$ cups	5 minutes	25 minutes	$1\frac{1}{4}$ cups
Each serving has:			
298 calories	8 g fat	1 g saturated fat	4 mg cholesterol
7 g fiber	192 mg sodium		

1 tsp. corn or canola oil

$\frac{1}{2}$ cup onion, chopped

1 clove garlic, minced

4 oz. mushrooms, chopped

$\frac{1}{2}$ cup steel-cut oats, uncooked

2 TB. white wine

$1\frac{3}{4}$ cups low-sodium chicken broth

$\frac{1}{2}$ cup fresh, cooked, or frozen thawed peas

$\frac{1}{8}$ tsp. ground black pepper

$\frac{1}{2}$ tsp. dried thyme (or 1 tsp. fresh)

1 TB. nonfat plain Greek-style yogurt

2 TB. Parmesan cheese

1. Heat corn oil in a $2\frac{1}{2}$-quart pot over medium-high heat; add onion and garlic and cook, stirring frequently, about 2 minutes.
2. Mix in mushrooms and steel-cut oats and cook another 2 minutes. Add white wine and 1 cup low-sodium chicken broth. Bring to a simmer, stirring occasionally. After 10 minutes, add remaining $\frac{3}{4}$ cup broth. Simmer an additional 10 minutes, stirring occasionally.
3. Stir in peas, black pepper, and thyme. Simmer 5 more minutes. Then take off heat and mix in nonfat Greek-style yogurt and Parmesan cheese. Texture should be creamy. Serve immediately.

DEFINITION

Risotto is an Italian rice dish that uses a special type of round short- or medium-grain rice (usually Arborio rice) cooked in a broth until rich and creamy, often with cheese and butter. Nowadays, however, it refers more to the technique than the rice and can feature any number of whole grains.

Indian Lentil Soup

Garam masala, a blend of different Indian spices, gives this lentil soup chock-full of vegetables its Eastern flavor.

Yield:	**Prep time:**	**Cook time:**	**Serving size:**
6 cups	20 minutes	40 minutes	1 cup
Each serving has:			
180 calories	3 g fat	1 g saturated fat	0 mg cholesterol
12 g fiber	175 mg sodium		

1 tsp. corn or vegetable oil

1 medium carrot (about 4 oz.), peeled and cut into 1-in. pieces

1 stalk celery, cut into 1-in. pieces

1 medium onion, cut into 1-in. pieces

1 garlic clove, minced

4 oz. mushrooms, sliced

2 medium tomatoes, diced

1 cup lentils, rinsed and picked through

5 cups low-sodium chicken or vegetable broth

$\frac{1}{4}$ tsp. sea salt or table salt

$\frac{1}{8}$ tsp. ground black pepper

2 tsp. garam masala

$\frac{1}{2}$ tsp. ground cumin

Fresh cilantro for garnish

1. Heat corn oil in a large saucepot over medium-high heat. Sauté carrot, celery, onion, and garlic for about 3 minutes. Add mushrooms and tomatoes, and sauté 1 more minute, stirring frequently.
2. Pour in lentils and low-sodium chicken broth, and stir in sea salt, black pepper, garam masala, and cumin. Bring to a boil and lower to a simmer. Cover. Simmer for 30 minutes.
3. To serve, sprinkle with fresh cilantro.

Fiber Boost: For a boost of fiber and texture, serve this lentil stew with brown basmati rice, about $\frac{1}{2}$ cup per serving.

HEALTHFUL LIVING

Lentils are brimming with fiber (1 cup cooked has nearly 16 grams of fiber), making them an ideal food for heart health. Foods high in soluble fiber are known for their cholesterol-reducing power. They're also good for weight loss, as they fill you up with few calories.

Stuffed Collard Greens

Although this stuffing contains lean ground beef, rice and vegetables are the main stars. Cooked in a rich tomato sauce, the greens become soft and tender. Make the rice and wheat berry mixture the night before, or use leftover cooked rice and grains, to save time.

Yield:	**Prep time:**	**Cook time:**	**Serving size:**
12 stuffed collard greens	25 minutes	1 hour	1 stuffed collard green
Each serving has:			
114 calories	2 g fat	1 g saturated fat	12 mg cholesterol
4 g fiber	114 mg sodium		

Filling:

1 large bunch collard greens (about 12 leaves), stems and stalks discarded

1 tsp. corn or canola oil

½ lb. ground beef (90 to 95 percent lean)

1 large carrot, peeled and diced into ¼-in. pieces

1 medium onion, diced into ¼-in. pieces

2 garlic cloves, minced

½ green bell pepper, diced into ¼-in. pieces

1 medium zucchini (4 oz.), diced into ¼-in. pieces

1 tsp. fennel seed, crushed

1 cup water

3 cups cooked brown rice and wheat berries*

½ tsp. kosher salt

¼ tsp. cayenne pepper

Sauce:

1 tsp. corn or canola oil

½ cup thinly sliced fennel bulb

½ cup chopped onion

3 cups crushed tomatoes plus 1 cup water *or* 1 (28-oz.) can crushed tomatoes with enough water added to make 4 cups

1 TB. granulated sugar

½ tsp dried basil (or 4 fresh basil leaves, chopped)

**To make rice–wheat berry mixture, cook ½ cup brown rice with ¼ cup wheat berries in 1¾ cups water over medium-high heat in medium saucepot covered for 1 hour (add more water, if needed).*

1. Prepare filling: Fill a large stock pot with water and bring to boil. Place collard leaves in boiling water for about 8 to 10 minutes or until tender, being careful not to tear leaves. Drain and rinse with cold water. Gently spread out on a large plate to cool. You can do this in two or three batches.

2. In a large sauté pan, heat corn oil over medium-high heat. Add lean ground beef and sauté, breaking up with a wooden spoon until you can't see any pink, about 3 minutes. Add carrot, onion, garlic, green bell pepper, and zucchini and cook another 3 or 4 minutes until soft.
3. Mix in fennel, water, cooked rice and wheat berries (or any leftover cooked whole grain), kosher salt, and cayenne pepper. Lower heat to medium, partially cover, and simmer about 5 or 6 minutes more until liquid is absorbed. Take off heat and set aside, uncovered, to cool.
4. Prepare sauce: In a medium saucepot, heat corn oil over medium-high heat, then sauté fennel and onion for about 3 or 4 minutes until vegetables begin to soften. Add crushed tomatoes and water, sugar, and basil. Cover and cook 30 minutes until all the flavors meld.
5. Preheat the oven to 350°F. To assemble, lay a collard leaf on a flat surface and place $^1/_2$ cup of rice mixture in center of leaf. Fold top over filling, fold both sides into the center, and roll into a cylinder. Repeat with remaining leaves.
6. Pour $^1/_2$ cup sauce on bottom of 9×13 roasting pan. Place any extra collard leaves on the bottom. Arrange stuffed collards seam side down on top of sauce. Pour remaining sauce over top of collards (be careful, it will be full). Cover with aluminum foil and bake in the oven for 40 to 45 minutes. Remove from the oven and serve immediately.

Fiber Boost: Add 2 cups cooked fresh or canned kidney beans to rice mixture filling, heat through, and stuff as directed in the recipe.

HEALTHFUL LIVING

Collard greens are a member of the cabbage family and are exceptionally high in vitamins A and K. They are also a rich source of fiber, vitamin C, and folate and are low in calories.

Asparagus with Sun-Dried Tomatoes, Quinoa, and Basmati Rice

Brown basmati rice and quinoa are cooked together and then tossed with sautéed asparagus, sun-dried tomatoes, mushrooms, and onions for a flavorful main dish that can served hot or cold.

Yield:	**Prep time:**	**Cook time:**	**Serving size:**
6 cups	10 minutes	45 minutes	1 cup
Each serving has:			
205 calories	5 g fat	1 g saturated fat	0 mg cholesterol
4 g fiber	171 mg sodium		

2 cups low-sodium chicken broth or vegetable broth

$\frac{1}{2}$ cup brown basmati rice

$\frac{1}{2}$ cup quinoa

1 tsp. corn or canola oil

3 oz. finely chopped red onion

1 garlic clove, minced

8 oz. asparagus, cut into $\frac{1}{2}$-in. pieces

8 oz. baby bella or cremini mushrooms, diced $\frac{1}{2}$ in.

$\frac{3}{4}$ cup sun-dried tomatoes, sliced into $\frac{1}{8}$-in. strips

$\frac{1}{4}$ cup chopped pistachios

2 TB. finely chopped oregano

2 TB. finely chopped parsley

$\frac{1}{8}$ tsp. ground black pepper

1. In a medium saucepot, bring low-sodium chicken broth to a boil. Add brown basmati rice. Cook, covered, for 25 minutes; then add quinoa and simmer, covered, for another 15 minutes. Set aside, covered, for 15 minutes. Then fluff with a fork.
2. In a large saucepan, heat corn oil over medium heat. When oil is hot, sauté red onion, garlic, asparagus, and baby bella mushrooms for about 4 minutes or until soft.
3. Add sun-dried tomatoes, pistachios, oregano, parsley, and black pepper. Gently mix in basmati rice and quinoa. Serve immediately.

Fiber Boost: Mix 1 cup asparagus mixture with $\frac{1}{2}$ cup of your favorite cooked beans (I like red beans). Serve.

HEALTHFUL LIVING

During peak season, asparagus can grow practically overnight. Some have been known to grow as much as 10 inches in a 24-hour period. Nutritionally, asparagus is high in folate, potassium, fiber, and vitamins A and C.

Rosemary Turkey and Oat Burger

Oats and grated zucchini add moisture to these turkey burgers. Tinged with apricot jam and whole-grain mustard, these burgers are spicy, sweet, and meaty.

Yield:	**Prep time:**	**Cook time:**	**Serving size:**
4 burgers	25 minutes	10 minutes	1 burger
Each serving has:			
146 calories	5 g fat	1 g saturated fat	44 mg cholesterol
2 g fiber	111 mg sodium		

8 oz. ground turkey

$\frac{1}{2}$ cup old-fashioned oats

2 tsp. whole-grain mustard

$\frac{1}{8}$ tsp. ground black pepper

$\frac{1}{4}$ cup green onions, finely chopped

2 TB. egg white

$\frac{1}{4}$ cup grated zucchini

$\frac{1}{2}$ tsp. fresh rosemary, finely chopped

1 tsp. garlic powder

1 tsp. Worcestershire sauce

1 TB. apricot jam

1. In a large bowl, mix ground turkey, old-fashioned oats, whole-grain mustard, black pepper, green onions, egg white, zucchini, rosemary, garlic powder, Worcestershire sauce, and apricot jam until well blended. Form into 4 ($3\frac{1}{2}$-oz.) patties and place in the refrigerator for 15 minutes.
2. Spray a large sauté pan with cooking spray and heat on medium-high. Place turkey burgers in the pan and cook about 5 to 6 minutes on each side. Or heat a grill to medium-high heat and spray turkey burgers with cooking spray. Place on the grill and let cook for 5 to 6 minutes on each side until done.
3. Serve plain in a salad or on a bun with your favorite toppings.

Fiber Boost: Serve these burgers on a whole-wheat pita topped with $\frac{1}{4}$ cup hummus (see Spicy Hummus in a Pita recipe in Chapter 19), lettuce, tomato, and cucumber.

HEART-SMART HABITS

To prevent lean turkey burgers from drying out, mix them with dried fruits; chopped or grated vegetables; salsa; tomato sauce; nuts; and any number of herbs, spices, and seasoning ingredients.

Chicken and Bean Burrito

Cooked chicken is tossed together with spicy salsa, beans, and corn and rolled into a whole-wheat tortilla in this simple, easy-to-make weeknight meal that comes together in minutes.

Yield:	**Prep time:**	**Cook time:**	**Serving size:**
4 burritos	10 minutes	8 minutes	1 burrito
Each serving has:			
277 calories	4 g fat	.4 g saturated fat	24 cholesterol
7 g fiber	399 mg sodium		

4 oz. boneless, skinless chicken breast, sliced into very thin strips

1 cup cooked red beans, any kind (if canned, drain and rinse)

1 cup corn, thawed from frozen or cooked from fresh

2 TB. chopped fresh cilantro

2 TB. nonfat plain Greek-style yogurt

2 TB. low-sodium salsa

4 (8-in.) whole-wheat flour tortillas

Toppings: nonfat yogurt, shredded lettuce, diced tomatoes

1. Spray a medium sauté pan with cooking spray and heat over medium-high heat until hot. Add chicken and cook, stirring frequently, for about 3 to 4 minutes until chicken is cooked through. Set aside to cool.
2. In a large bowl, stir together red beans, corn, cilantro, nonfat Greek-style yogurt, and low-sodium salsa. Gently mix in cooked chicken.
3. Spread 8-inch whole-wheat tortilla on a flat surface. Place ½ cup of chicken and bean mixture in center of tortilla. Fold up one side to center, then fold in two ends and roll up to form a burrito. Repeat for next 3 burritos.
4. Serve immediately with a dollop of nonfat yogurt, shredded lettuce, and diced tomatoes. Burritos will keep in the refrigerator for 3 days; reheat in the microwave or oven.

Fiber Boost: To make these burritos even higher in fiber, add ¼ to ½ cup cooked brown rice, wild rice, or wild rice blend (per serving) to the bean mixture right before wrapping the burrito.

GOTCHA!

Nearly all the fat in chicken is found in the skin. In fact, by removing the skin, you remove more than half the fat. Consider that a 3½-ounce piece of chicken breast with the skin has 8 grams of fat and nearly 200 calories, while the same amount of white-meat chicken without the skin has only 3½ grams of fat and about 165 calories.

Buffalo Tacos

If you've never tasted buffalo, it's definitely worth a try. Leaner than beef, buffalo cooks fast and has a meaty, robust flavor that's not gamey. The filling for this taco is done in less than 20 minutes.

Yield:	**Prep time:**	**Cook time:**	**Serving size:**
8 tacos	5 minutes	15 minutes	2 tacos
Each serving has:			
301 calories	8 g fat	2 g saturated fat	32 mg cholesterol
6 g fiber	428 mg sodium		

- 1 dried ancho pepper, seeded and stem removed, cut into pieces
- 1 tsp. chipotle chile powder
- 1 tsp. ground cumin
- 1 tsp. Mexican oregano (or any kind of oregano)
- $\frac{1}{8}$ tsp. ground black pepper
- 1 TB. corn or canola oil
- $\frac{1}{2}$ small onion, finely chopped
- 2 garlic cloves, minced
- 8 oz. grass-fed ground bison
- $\frac{1}{2}$ cup tomato purée
- $\frac{1}{2}$ cup water
- $\frac{1}{2}$ cup cooked red beans, drained and rinsed
- 2 tsp. teff flour or buckwheat flour
- $\frac{1}{2}$ tsp. sea salt
- 8 (6-in.) corn tortillas
- Toppings: shredded lettuce, diced tomatoes, diced cucumber, nonfat yogurt

1. Place ancho pepper, chipotle chile powder, cumin, Mexican oregano, and black pepper in a spice or coffee grinder and grind to a fine powder (about 1 minute).
2. Heat corn oil in a medium sauté pan over medium-high heat and add onion, garlic, and spice mixture. Cook for about 2 minutes, stirring frequently. Add bison and stir for another 2 minutes until meat browns.
3. Mix in tomato purée and water. Reduce heat to a simmer, and simmer, covered, for 5 minutes. Stir in red beans and teff flour. Simmer, covered, another 5 minutes. Add sea salt.
4. To serve, place $\frac{1}{4}$ cup bison mixture on each corn tortilla. Top with shredded lettuce, diced tomatoes, diced cucumber, and a dollop of nonfat yogurt.

HEART-SMART HABITS

When choosing ground bison, be sure to read the label. Always look for grass-fed over regular or corn-fed bison (another term is grain-finished); it's lower in fat.

Mahi-Mahi over Farro with Butternut Squash

Here, lemony mahi-mahi is served on a bed of pesto-flavored *farro* flecked with butternut squash. If you want to add more color, try throwing in a chopped steamed green like Swiss chard or kale.

Yield:	Prep time:	Cook time:	Serving size:
5 cups farro and 12 ounces mahi-mahi	10 minutes	40 minutes	$1\frac{1}{4}$ cups farro and 3 ounces mahi-mahi
Each serving has:			
368 calories	10 g fat	1 g saturated fat	61 mg cholesterol
7 g fiber	367 mg sodium		

$3\frac{1}{2}$ cups water

1 cup farro

2 tsp. corn or canola oil

$\frac{1}{2}$ cup red onion, finely diced

$2\frac{1}{2}$ cups butternut squash, cut into $\frac{1}{4}$-in. dice

4 tsp. prepared pesto

4 (3-oz.) boneless, skinless mahi-mahi fillets

2 tsp. lemon juice

1 tsp. lemon zest

Salt and pepper to taste

1. Preheat the oven to 500°F.
2. In a medium saucepan, heat $2\frac{1}{2}$ cups water to boiling. Add farro. Bring to a boil, reduce heat to a simmer, and cook, covered, about 30 minutes until water is absorbed and farro is tender.
3. When farro has cooked for about 20 minutes, begin rest of the recipe. In another saucepan, heat 1 teaspoon corn oil over medium-high heat. Add red onion and sauté for 2 minutes. Add butternut squash and sauté 1 more minute. Add remaining 1 cup water and simmer on low, covered, for 8 minutes or until squash is tender. When squash and vegetables are done, gently mix into farro mixture along with pesto and set aside covered.
4. Place mahi-mahi on a baking pan sprayed with cooking spray. Sprinkle fish with lemon juice, lemon zest, and remaining 1 teaspoon corn oil. Sprinkle with salt and pepper.

5. Cook fish for 5 to 7 minutes until it flakes easily with a fork.
6. To serve, place fish fillet over $1\frac{1}{4}$ cup of butternut squash–farro mixture.

DEFINITION

Farro (or **grano farro**) is an ancient strain of wheat that's popular in Italy. It is used to make bread and small pasta and is common in soups and side dishes. Look for whole-grain farro.

Oven-Fried Catfish with Cornmeal Cakes

This oven-fried catfish is so crispy, you'd never know it wasn't fried. Drizzled with some honey and pecans and served over cornmeal cakes, it's divine!

Yield:	**Prep time:**	**Cook time:**	**Serving size:**
6 catfish fillets and 12 cornmeal cakes	10 minutes	50 minutes	1 catfish fillet and 2 cornmeal cakes
Each serving has:			
340 calories	14 g fat	2 g saturated fat	40 mg cholesterol
4 g fiber	528 mg sodium		

3½ cups water

1¼ tsp. kosher salt

½ cup plus ⅓ cup coarse cornmeal

¾ cup chopped green onion

¾ tsp. cayenne pepper

½ cup white whole-wheat flour

½ cup corn flour

1 tsp. onion powder

1 tsp. garlic powder

1 tsp. paprika

¼ tsp. freshly ground black pepper

1 tsp. ground thyme

½ cup egg substitute

6 (3-oz.) boneless, skinless catfish fillets

1 TB. soft margarine

1 TB. honey

1 TB. water

1 TB. pecans, chopped

1. Preheat the oven to 450°F.
2. In a large saucepot, heat water to boiling. Add ½ teaspoon kosher salt. Slowly pour in coarse cornmeal in a thin stream, whisking constantly with a wire whisk so it doesn't get lumpy. Water should be continuously boiling. Once you have added all the cornmeal, switch to a wooden spoon, mixing frequently to prevent sticking on the bottom and the sides. Cornmeal will continue to pop and boil. Cook, uncovered, for 30 minutes, stirring frequently. Five minutes before cornmeal is done, mix in chopped green onion and ½ teaspoon cayenne pepper or as much as you like. Once cornmeal is cooked, pour it into a loaf pan, smooth top, and let cool.
3. While cornmeal is cooling, in a medium bowl, mix together white whole-wheat flour, corn flour, onion powder, garlic powder, paprika, black pepper, thyme, remaining ¾ teaspoon kosher salt, and remaining ¼ teaspoon cayenne pepper until well blended.

4. In another separate bowl, beat egg substitute.
5. To assemble, dip catfish fillets in egg substitute, then flour mixture, then egg substitute, then flour again.
6. Spray a cookie sheet with cooking spray. Lay fish on the cookie sheet and spray tops with cooking spray. Place in the oven and cook 10 to 12 minutes. Gently turn over with a spatula and cook another 5 minutes.
7. Slice cooled cornmeal into 12 slices about $\frac{1}{2}$ inch thick. After cornmeal is sliced, heat a medium sauté pan over medium-high heat. Add margarine, honey, water, and pecans to pan. Swirl it around to melt.
8. To serve, place two slices of cornmeal on a plate, top with one catfish fillet, and drizzle with 1 tablespoon honey-margarine and water mixture and 1 teaspoon pecans.

HEART-SMART HABITS

U.S.-farmed catfish is sustainably raised in environmentally sound inland ponds in the southeastern United States (Mississippi is the number one state). Catfish tastes mild and sweet (not fishy) and is low in fat. Avoid catfish raised in China, as it may contain contaminants.

Flavor Boosters

Chapter **17**

In This Chapter

- Zesty marinades and vinaigrettes
- Sassy bean spreads and sauces
- New ways with tofu
- Saltless spice blends

Welcome to the wonderful world of herbs, spices, and citrus. These foods boost flavor without relying on salt and saturated fat like butter or cream, ideal for the TLC diet. They also provide great diversity and excitement to any meal, not to mention a healthful dose of plant antioxidants. In fact, ounce for ounce, herbs and spices are nature's most concentrated source of these beneficial plant compounds.

But it is for their distinct taste and vibrant color that herbs and spices are most prized. As you get more familiar with them and get accustomed to using them, you'll begin to recognize all the culinary opportunities they offer.

The recipes in this chapter use both fresh herbs and dried spices. Herbs are the aromatic green leaves of a plant and include parsley, basil, cilantro, and oregano, to name a few. Spices come from plants, too—usually the dried bark, root, seeds, buds, or berries—and are whole, crushed, or ground. They naturally contain no salt, sugar, or fat.

In the kitchen, their value is in their versatility as well as taste. Consider parsley, which can be combined with cilantro for a Mexican slant, added to basil for something Italian, or mixed with fresh fennel leaves for a more French Provençal flair. Not only are the individual ingredients flexible (in the Orange-Lime Marinade, if you don't have oregano, you can substitute cilantro or parsley), but the recipes are as well.

All of them have at least two culinary applications. The Corn-Olive-Tomato Salsa, for example, is great as an accompaniment to broiled salmon or grilled pork, works as a topping for a bean burrito, and can be tossed with greens as an interesting salad dressing.

Using herbs and spices is also fast and easy. With just a few exceptions, most recipes use only a handful of ingredients and can be whipped up within a few minutes in a food processor. Others, like the Red Pepper Tofu, can easily be made the night before.

Think of these recipes as guidelines you can adapt or change to fit your own individual taste or style. Don't like spicy foods? Omit the red pepper. Like things hot? Bump it up a notch and double the amount. The choice is yours. Who says healthful foods have to be boring or bland? Not these!

Corn-Olive-Tomato Salsa

In this version of a salsa, colorful sweet corn and tomatoes are tossed with the bright, fresh flavors of a cilantro-parsley-green olive sauce, then finished with a splash of tart lime juice and a jalapeño for some heat.

Yield:	**Prep time:**	**Serving size:**	
2 cups	10 minutes	$\frac{1}{4}$ cup	
Each serving has:			
55 calories	4 g fat	0 g saturated fat	0 mg cholesterol
1 g fiber	33 mg sodium		

$\frac{1}{2}$ cup firmly packed cilantro, leaves and stems

$\frac{1}{4}$ cup firmly packed parsley, leaves and stems

1 garlic clove

5 green stuffed pimento olives, sliced in half

2 TB. canola or corn oil

2 TB. white vinegar

1 medium tomato, seeded and diced into $\frac{1}{2}$-in. pieces

1 cup thawed-from-frozen or fresh-cooked corn

1 TB. finely minced jalapeño

$\frac{1}{2}$ medium lime

1. In the bowl of a small food chopper or food processor, place cilantro, parsley, garlic, pimento olives, canola oil, and white vinegar. Pulse for about 30 seconds until herbs are finely chopped and olives are slightly chunky.
2. In a medium bowl, toss together tomato, corn, and jalapeño. Pour in cilantro-parsley sauce. Right before serving, squeeze $\frac{1}{2}$ lime over top of salsa and gently mix. Serve as an accompaniment to fish, chicken, or pork; use as a topping for a bean burrito; mix into rice or another grain like quinoa; or toss with greens for a spicy salad dressing.

HEART-SMART HABITS

Though olives are considered a high-sodium, high-fat food, when used as a seasoning ingredient in small amounts, they can easily be included on the TLC diet. Plus, the type of fat found in olives, monounsaturated and polyunsaturated, is the good kind.

Spinach Tofu Pesto

Mild spinach and tangy arugula are puréed with sliced almonds and garlic for a flavorful pesto. To keep the fat content down, soft tofu replaces much of the olive oil in this recipe, creating a smooth, rich taste and creamy consistency.

Yield:	**Prep time:**	**Serving size:**	
1¼ cups	5 minutes	¼ cup	
Each serving has:			
75 calories	4 g fat	1 g saturated fat	0 mg cholesterol
1 g fiber	109 mg sodium		

- 2 cups packed spinach
- 1 cup packed arugula
- 1 garlic clove
- 1 TB. sliced almonds
- ¾ cup soft tofu (about 4 oz.)
- 2 TB. olive oil (or any vegetable oil)
- ¼ tsp. kosher salt
- Dash freshly ground black pepper

1. In the bowl of a large food processor, place spinach, arugula, garlic, almonds, soft tofu, olive oil, kosher salt, and black pepper. Purée for about 30 seconds or until smooth.
2. Serve alongside chicken or fish, or with roasted or grilled vegetables, whole-wheat pasta, or any whole-grain mixture.

HEALTHFUL LIVING

Leafy greens like spinach and arugula are nutrient dense, meaning they are high in nutrients and low in calories. Some of the most noteworthy are beta-carotene, vitamin C, vitamin K, folate, and the phytochemicals zeaxanthin and lutein, which protect eye health.

Orange-Lime Marinade

This citrusy marinade combines sweet orange juice with tart lime juice and a touch of maple syrup. The combination is more common than you think. Zest makes the flavors pop, while cumin and fresh oregano give it a Cuban flair.

Yield:	**Prep time:**	**Serving size:**	
3/4 cup	5 minutes	1 tablespoon	
Each serving has:			
11 calories	0 g fat	0 g saturated fat	0 mg cholesterol
0 g fiber	25 mg sodium		

Zest from 1 large orange (about 1 TB.)

1/2 cup orange juice

Zest from 1 lime (about 2 tsp.)

Juice from 1 lime (about 2 tsp.)

1 TB. maple syrup

1/2 tsp. ground cumin

2 TB. oregano, finely chopped (can substitute cilantro or parsley)

1/8 tsp. sea salt or table salt

1/4 tsp. freshly ground black pepper

1. In a small bowl, mix orange zest, orange juice, lime zest, lime juice, maple syrup, cumin, oregano, sea salt, and black pepper with a wire whisk until well blended.
2. Use as a marinade for chicken or fish or as a sauce for vegetables or grains.

Variation: For **Orange-Lime Salad Dressing,** blend in 1 tablespoon vegetable oil to entire recipe.

GOTCHA!

Some conventionally grown citrus like lemons and limes have a waxy coating to protect them during shipping, so if you're going to use the zest, this is one time where using organically grown (and wax-free) produce is important.

Red Pepper Tofu

Dried and crumbled *tofu* takes the place of a salty cheese high in saturated fat. Pressing tofu removes the water and gives it a chewy texture that is similar to meat or chicken. Letting the tofu sit overnight gives it time to absorb the flavors of oregano, basil, and lemon zest. The rice vinegar gives it a sharp, tangy taste not unlike feta.

Yield:	**Prep time:**	**Marinade time:**	**Serving size:**
1 cup	1 hour, 5 minutes	Overnight	2 tablespoons
Each serving has:			
14 calories	.4 g fat	0 g saturated fat	0 mg cholesterol
0 g fiber	44 mg sodium		

- 6 oz. firm tofu, cut in ½-in. slices
- 2 TB. rice vinegar
- ¼ cup diced red bell pepper, raw or roasted from a jar
- ¼ tsp. dried oregano
- ¼ tsp. dried basil
- ¼ tsp. lemon zest
- ⅛ tsp. red pepper flakes (optional)
- ⅛ tsp. kosher salt
- Dash freshly ground black pepper

1. To squeeze water out of tofu, place tofu slices on a wire rack, cover with paper towels, and place a clean cutting board over top. Place several heavy books on top of the cutting board. Keep tofu like this for about 30 to 45 minutes, changing the paper towels often.
2. When tofu is dry, remove from the rack and crumble into a small bowl. Add rice vinegar, red bell pepper, oregano, basil, lemon zest, red pepper flakes (if using), kosher salt, and black pepper. Gently toss together.
3. Store in an airtight container in the refrigerator at least 8 hours or overnight, to allow flavors to develop.
4. Serve tofu in place of feta on top of salads, stir into rice dishes, and sprinkle on top of vegetables.

DEFINITION

Tofu is a mildly flavored food made from pressed soybeans and formed into a smooth curd. It comes in three types: soft, best for soups, dips, and desserts; firm or regular, good as an all-purpose tofu for stir-fry and mixed dishes; and extra-firm, good for grills, tofu steaks, or kebobs. Tofu is famous for taking on flavors.

Honey Avocado Cilantro Vinaigrette

Finely diced avocado gives this bright green cilantro dressing a creamy taste, while honey and red pepper flakes add sweet-spicy notes. Enhanced with lemon juice and garlic, this is one dressing you'll be making over and over again.

Yield:	**Prep time:**	**Serving size:**	
1 cup	10 minutes	1 tablespoon	
Each serving has:			
44 calories	2.7 g fat	.3 g saturated fat	0 mg cholesterol
.5 g fiber	38 mg sodium		

2 cups packed cilantro
¼ cup rice vinegar
¼ cup honey
3 garlic cloves
¼ tsp. sea salt or table salt
⅛ tsp. freshly ground black pepper
2 TB. corn, olive, or vegetable oil
1 TB. lemon juice
¼ tsp. red pepper flakes
½ avocado, peeled and cut into ¼-in. dice

1. Place cilantro, rice vinegar, honey, garlic, sea salt, black pepper, corn oil, lemon juice, and red pepper flakes in the bowl of a food processor and purée for 30 to 40 seconds until smooth.
2. Pour into a bowl and gently mix in avocado.
3. Use this as a salad dressing for mixed greens, whole grains, or bean salads.

GOTCHA!

When it comes to salad dressings, always choose oil-and-vinegar dressings (or make your own) over premade bottled salad dressing. The prepared dressings are usually loaded with salt, sugar, and fat (particularly if they're creamy varieties), not to mention artificial flavors and ingredients like dyes.

Peanut Grapefruit Dressing

Peanuts and grapefruit may seem like an odd combination, but they work beautifully in this Asian-inspired soy sauce–based dressing. Chunks of grapefruit give texture and a boost of vitamin C, while peanut butter makes the dressing creamy and rich. Goes great as a marinade or dressing for chicken with noodles.

Yield:	**Prep time:**	**Serving size:**	
1 cup	10 minutes	1 tablespoon	
Each serving has:			
26 calories	1.6 g fat	.2 g saturated fat	0 mg cholesterol
0 g fiber	72 mg sodium		

2 TB. plus 1 tsp. rice wine vinegar

2 TB. low-sodium soy sauce

1 TB. honey

4 TB. water

1 TB. all-natural unsweetened smooth peanut butter

2 tsp. peanut, corn, or vegetable oil

1 tsp. sesame oil

1 pink or white grapefruit sectioned and diced (about $\frac{3}{4}$ cup), juice reserved

1 TB. finely chopped unsalted roasted peanuts

1. In a small bowl, whisk together rice wine vinegar, low-sodium soy sauce, honey, water, peanut butter, peanut oil, sesame oil, and 2 tablespoons reserved grapefruit juice until smooth.
2. Stir in grapefruit pieces and roasted peanuts.
3. Serve on salad greens, as a marinade for chicken or fish, or over top of Chinese noodles and vegetables.

HEALTHFUL LIVING

To section a grapefruit, place the fruit on a flat, clean work surface. Cut off both ends and place the flat side down. Next, cut off the outside skin and white pith, leaving only the fruit. Then cut the fruit on both sides along each section to the center, like a triangle, and pop out the fruit section. To save the juice, once finished, squeeze the grapefruit membranes over a bowl. You should get about 2 tablespoons of juice from one section of grapefruit.

TLC Tapenade

This tapenade is more like a red pepper hummus with chopped kalamata olives. The recipe calls for parsley, oregano, and fennel, giving it a slightly licorice flavor, but you can use any herb combination you like.

Yield: 1 cup	**Prep time:** 5 minutes	**Serving size:** 2 tablespoons	
Each serving has:			
42 calories	2.6 g fat	.2 g saturated fat	0 mg cholesterol
1 g fiber	18 mg sodium		

- ½ cup cooked fresh or canned chickpeas (if using canned, drain and rinse)
- 1 TB. lemon juice
- 1 TB. olive, corn, or vegetable oil
- 1 TB. water
- ½ large red bell pepper, peeled, seeded, and roasted (can be from jar)
- ¼ cup packed roughly chopped fresh parsley
- ¼ cup packed roughly chopped fresh oregano
- ¼ cup packed roughly chopped fresh fennel leaves
- 5 kalamata olives, roughly chopped

1. Place chickpeas, lemon juice, olive oil, water, red bell pepper, parsley, oregano, and fennel in a food processor bowl and process for 20 to 30 seconds, scraping down the sides of the bowl frequently so everything is chopped.
2. Once mixture is smooth, pour into a bowl and stir in kalamata olives.
3. Use as a dip or spread for vegetables, or toss with brown rice or quinoa and broccoli or spinach.

HEART-SMART HABITS

Canned beans are notoriously high in sodium. To cut the salt, drain and rinse canned beans. This can cut sodium by 40 percent, dropping a ½-cup serving of chickpeas from 360 mg sodium to 216 mg sodium.

Edamame Basil Spread

In this creamy spread, mildly sweet *edamame* beans pair with cooling yogurt and sweet basil with just a hint of coriander and tart lemon zest. This spread is perfect paired with a spicy Indian cuisine or a meaty fish like mahi-mahi.

Yield:	**Prep time:**	**Serving size:**	
$1\frac{1}{4}$ cups	10 minutes	$\frac{1}{4}$ cup	
Each serving has:			
52 calories	1.7 g fat	.2 g saturated fat	0 mg cholesterol
2 g fiber	107 mg sodium		

1 cup frozen-thawed edamame beans or baby lima beans

$\frac{1}{4}$ cup shredded basil leaves

$\frac{1}{2}$ cup nonfat or low-fat plain yogurt

1 tsp. ground coriander

$\frac{1}{4}$ tsp. kosher salt

$\frac{1}{8}$ tsp. freshly ground black pepper

Zest of one lemon (about 2 tsp.)

2 TB. water

1. Cook edamame according to the package directions, omitting salt and butter. Once cooked, drain and rinse under warm water. Place edamame, basil, nonfat yogurt, coriander, kosher salt, black pepper, and lemon zest in a food processor and process for about 30 to 40 seconds until smooth and creamy. Add water if necessary for a thinner consistency.
2. Pour into a bowl and serve. Use a dollop on soup or salads with fish or chicken, on sandwiches, and paired with spicy foods like Dahl.

DEFINITION

Edamame are fresh green soybeans; they taste sweet and clean. Although you can find them shelled, they are most often sold frozen in their inedible pod.

Spicy Italian Seasoning Blend

Make a big batch of this all-purpose seasoning blend, and you'll find yourself using it in everything. A mixture of popular dried Italian spices like basil, oregano, and parsley, it is most welcome in the winter, when fresh herbs are hard to find. If you don't like spicy, omit the red pepper flakes.

Yield:	**Prep time:**	**Serving size:**	
4 tablespoons	5 minutes	1 teaspoon	
Each serving has:			
5 calories	0 g fat	0 g saturated fat	0 mg cholesterol
.2 g fiber	1 mg sodium		

1 TB. minced dried onion

1 TB. dried parsley flakes

1 TB. minced dried garlic

1 tsp. dried oregano leaves

1 tsp. dried basil leaves

$\frac{1}{2}$ tsp. dried red pepper flakes (optional)

1. Mix dried onion, parsley, garlic, oregano, basil, and red pepper flakes (if using) in a small bowl. Pour into a clean, dry jar and store in your spice cabinet. This will keep for a year or longer.
2. Serve on vegetables; in sauces; on garlic bread; in grain mixtures; and on meat, fish, or poultry.

GOTCHA!

Beware of prepared spice blends. Many are laced with salt and sugar. Read the label before buying.

Fennel-Coriander Spice Blend

Fennel and coriander are known as sweet spices because they are often used in place of cinnamon in desserts. Here they are mixed with allspice and black pepper for a blend that can be either sweet or savory.

Yield:	**Prep time:**	**Serving size:**	
5 tablespoons	5 minutes	1 teaspoon	
Each serving has:			
5 calories	0 g fat	0 g saturated fat	0 mg cholesterol
0 g fiber	1 mg sodium		

3 TB. coriander seed

1 TB. fennel seed

$\frac{1}{2}$ tsp ground allspice

1 tsp. freshly ground black pepper

1. Place coriander and fennel in a spice grinder or coffee grinder and grind until smooth (about 20 seconds). Add allspice and black pepper, and mix thoroughly. Store in a clean glass jar in your spice cabinet. This will keep for 6 months to a year or longer.
2. Use on fish (excellent on salmon), meat, chicken, and vegetables. You can also add to baked items in place of cinnamon for an unusual and exotic flavor.

HEALTHFUL LIVING

Allspice is a three-in-one spice that tastes like cinnamon, nutmeg, and cloves all rolled into one. It is best bought whole as small, dry black berries and freshly ground as needed.

Soups, Pizzas, and Salads

Chapter 18

In This Chapter

- Super suppertime soups
- Pizza you can feel good about
- Great green salads
- Making main dish salads a snap

Soups, pizzas, and salads are great ways to increase your vegetable, bean, and grain intake without feeling like you're missing out on anything. Plus, they're easy to make, inexpensive, and extremely versatile. Each one also has its own unique culinary qualities that contribute to good health.

Consider soup, for example. Typical soups, like cream of broccoli or tomato, are laden with heavy cream, cheese, and salt—a nutritional nightmare. TLC soups are broth-based, go easy on the salt (with low-sodium or homemade stock), and are loaded with beans and vegetables. The result is a low-calorie, nutrient-dense soup that's big on flavor, filling and satisfying, and low in fat—just taste my Zucchini Minestrone soup to find out. The beauty of soup, too, is its forgiving nature. Don't have zucchini? Use butternut squash or broccoli. Missing chickpeas? Substitute red beans or kidney beans.

When it comes to salad, skip the bacon and the bottled salad dressing. Instead, focus on vegetables like carrots, cauliflower, and celery, and make your own dressing, like the creamy yogurt dressing in the Tuna and Apple Salad or the orange-honey vinaigrette for the Beet and Orange Salad. You can mix and match these salad dressings with any combination of vegetables, greens, and beans. Don't be alarmed to see a few robust cheeses, either. Low-fat versions of feta and blue cheese are used sparingly to add flavor with minimal fat. Perfect when you're on the go, these salads are great as a side, or up the portion and feature them as a main entrée. They're super.

Pizzas can be a nutritious and delicious healthful main meal, if you think outside the box. Forget the high-sodium sauce, heavy cheese, and fatty meats. Build your own pizzas using flavored olive oil or hummus as a base. You don't have to stick with traditional vegetable toppings, either. My Hummus Pizza with Sun-Dried Tomatoes is topped with red onion and cooked Swiss chard. You could also use sautéed spinach and a few black olives in place of the Swiss chard and sun-dried tomatoes, or maybe some roasted red bell peppers and onions. The sky's the limit when it comes to pizza combinations. In fact, all the dishes featured in this chapter—soups, salads, and pizza—are meant to inspire you and encourage you to try new vegetables or flavors. Just use your imagination.

Navy Bean Soup

Kale gives this classic tomato-based navy bean soup an antioxidant boost, as well as a splash of color. Flavored with fresh thyme and a hint of maple syrup, serve this hearty soup when the weather turns cold.

Yield:	**Prep time:**	**Cook time:**	**Serving size:**
10 cups	20 minutes	$2\frac{1}{2}$ hours	1 cup
Each serving has:			
211 calories	2 g fat	.4 g saturated fat	0 mg cholesterol
13 g fiber	188 mg sodium		

1 tsp. corn or canola oil

1 garlic clove, minced

1 medium stalk celery, $\frac{1}{4}$ in. diced

1 medium carrot, peeled $\frac{1}{4}$ in. diced

1 medium onion, $\frac{1}{4}$ in. diced

4 cups low-sodium chicken broth

3 cups water

1 lb. dried navy beans, presoaked overnight (see sidebar for fast method)

3 large bay leaves

1 tsp. chopped fresh thyme

2 TB. maple syrup

$1\frac{1}{2}$ cups crushed tomatoes

$\frac{1}{4}$ tsp. freshly ground black pepper

$\frac{1}{2}$ tsp. kosher salt

2 cups finely chopped kale

1. In a large saucepan, heat corn oil over medium heat. Add garlic, celery, carrot, and onion and sauté for 3 minutes until vegetables begin to soften.
2. Add low-sodium chicken broth, water, navy beans, and bay leaves. Bring to a boil. Stir in thyme, maple syrup, tomatoes, black pepper, and kosher salt. Bring back to a boil. Reduce heat to simmer for $1\frac{1}{2}$ hours.
3. Stir in chopped kale, and simmer for 30 minutes. Soup is done when beans are soft and flavors have blended. Serve immediately.

HEART-SMART HABITS

Forget to soak your beans overnight? No problem. Simply pour beans into a saucepan with enough water to cover. Heat on high until beans come to a gentle boil (beans will start to float to the top). Boil for 2 minutes. Take beans off the heat, cover, and let soak in water 1 to 2 hours or more (the longer, the better). Then cook as you would normally.

Tomato Basil White Bean Soup

This classic tomato soup is kicked up a notch with fresh basil and chunky *cannellini beans.* Add a crusty whole-wheat bread or a light salad, and you have a quick weekday supper.

Yield:	**Prep time:**	**Cook time:**	**Serving size:**
4 cups	15 minutes	20 minutes	1 cup
Each serving has:			
186 calories	2 g fat	0 g saturated fat	0 mg cholesterol
8 g fiber	277 mg sodium		

1 tsp. corn or canola oil

$\frac{1}{2}$ cup white onion, $\frac{1}{4}$ in. diced

$\frac{1}{4}$ cup celery, $\frac{1}{4}$ in. diced

1 garlic clove, minced

$\frac{1}{4}$ cup chopped basil

1 (14-oz.) can or box crushed tomatoes (about 2 cups)

1 (15-oz.) can cannellini beans, drained and rinsed (about $1\frac{3}{4}$ cups cooked)

1 cup low-sodium chicken or vegetable broth or water

$\frac{1}{4}$ tsp. kosher salt

$\frac{1}{8}$ tsp. freshly ground black pepper

1. Heat corn oil over medium-high heat in a large saucepan. Add white onion, celery, and garlic and sauté for about 1 to 2 minutes, stirring constantly, until vegetables begin to soften.
2. Stir in basil, tomatoes, cannellini beans, low-sodium chicken broth, kosher salt, and black pepper. Bring to a simmer and cover. Simmer for 15 minutes until vegetables are tender and flavors blend. Serve immediately.

DEFINITION

Cannellini beans are often called white kidney beans because these large beans have a kidney-bean shape and are creamy inside. They have a mild taste and thin skin.

Zucchini Minestrone

In Italy, *minestrone* means any thick vegetable soup with pasta. This version is loaded with zucchini, carrots, cabbage, tomato, and white beans. Farro is a chewy Italian grain that takes the place of pasta.

Yield: 10 cups	**Prep time:** 10 minutes	**Cook time:** 50 minutes	**Serving size:** 1 cup
Each serving has:			
122 calories	2 g fat	.4 g saturated fat	0 mg cholesterol
5 g fiber	167 mg sodium		

1 tsp. canola or corn oil
1 stalk celery, small dice
1 medium onion, small dice
1 medium zucchini, small dice
1 large carrot, small dice
4 oz. cabbage, small dice
1 garlic clove, minced
1 medium tomato, small dice
1 low-sodium 15-ounce can white beans, drained and rinsed (or $1\frac{1}{2}$ cups cooked chickpeas)
7 cups low-sodium chicken or vegetable broth
$\frac{1}{2}$ cup farro
3 large basil leaves, chopped
$\frac{1}{4}$ cup Italian parsley, loosely packed, roughly chopped
$\frac{1}{2}$ tsp. kosher salt
$\frac{1}{4}$ tsp. freshly ground black pepper

1. Heat canola oil in a large 3-quart stockpot over medium heat. Add celery, onion, zucchini, carrot, cabbage, and garlic. Cook for about 4 minutes, covered, stirring occasionally.
2. Mix in tomato, white beans, low-sodium chicken broth, farro, basil, Italian parsley, kosher salt, and black pepper. Bring to a boil. Reduce to a simmer and cook with the cover ajar for 40 minutes until vegetables are tender. Serve immediately.

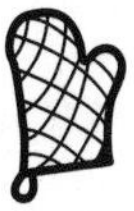

HEART-SMART HABITS

Broth-based and tomato-based soups are two of the best foods to eat for cutting calories. These soups fill you up without a lot of calories so you eat less. They can also help you keep the weight from coming back. Studies done by Barbara Rolls at Penn State found dieters who regularly ate low-calorie, dense foods like soup kept the weight off better than dieters who didn't.

Easy Whole-Wheat Pizza Dough

This dough is so easy to make, even a novice can do it. It has a superb nutty and yeasty flavor, with a light and airy texture.

Yield:	**Prep time:**	**Cook time:**	**Serving size:**
2 pizza doughs (1 pizza yields 12 slices)	15 minutes, plus 1 hour rising time	15 minutes	1 slice
Each serving has:			
74 calories	2 g fat	.2 g saturated fat	0 mg cholesterol
1.3 g fiber	98 mg sodium		

- $1\frac{1}{3}$ cups warm water
- 1 pkg. yeast ($2\frac{1}{4}$ tsp.)
- $1\frac{3}{4}$ cups whole-wheat flour (or white whole-wheat flour)
- $1\frac{1}{2}$ cups all-purpose flour
- 1 tsp. sea salt or table salt
- 3 TB. olive or vegetable oil

1. In a large bowl, mix warm water and yeast. Let sit for about 3 minutes. Add whole-wheat flour, all-purpose flour, and sea salt. Mix, then gradually drizzle in olive oil.
2. Knead on a well-floured board for about 8 minutes until dough is smooth and elastic.
3. Spray or oil a big bowl with cooking spray, and rub dough with oil or spray with cooking spray. Place in a bowl, cover with a dish towel, and let rise for 1 hour until dough is doubled in size.
4. Punch down dough and shape into pizza.

Variation: You can also do this whole process in a high-speed stand-up mixer with a dough hook. Place warm water, yeast, whole-wheat flour, all-purpose flour, and sea salt in a bowl and mix on high speed. Gradually add olive oil and mix for about 4 or 5 minutes until dough is smooth and elastic.

HEART-SMART HABITS

Make a double batch of this dough, and after it has risen, place it in a plastic bag and freeze. Thaw it out to room temperature, then shape it and let it rest for 20 minutes before baking.

Hummus Pizza with Sun-Dried Tomatoes

Pizza dough brushed with a rosemary-garlic oil and then baked to give it a crisp crunch is the base for this pizza, which is spread with *hummus* and sun-dried tomatoes. It's topped with Swiss chard to give it some color and extra nutrients.

Yield:	**Prep time:**	**Cook time:**	**Serving size:**
1 pizza (12 slices)	25 minutes	15 minutes	2 slices
Each serving has:			
192 calories	7 g fat	.7 g saturated fat	0 mg cholesterol
3.8 g fiber	335 mg sodium		

½ recipe for Easy Whole-Wheat Pizza Dough (see previous recipe) or 1 lb. pkg. frozen whole-wheat pizza dough, thawed

2 tsp. canola or olive oil

1 clove garlic, crushed

1 tsp. fresh rosemary, minced

½ cup slivered sun-dried tomatoes

½ cup slivered or chopped Swiss chard, spinach, or kale

¼ cup store-bought or homemade hummus (see Spicy Hummus in a Pita recipe in Chapter 19)

2 TB. chopped red onion

1. Heat the oven to 375°F.
2. Roll out Easy Whole-Wheat Pizza Dough in 12×12 square, and place on a pizza stone or cookie sheet sprayed with cooking spray. Let rise for about 15 minutes.
3. While Easy Whole-Wheat Pizza Dough is rising, place canola oil, garlic, and rosemary in a small glass container and microwave for about 30 to 40 seconds until oil is fragrant, stirring two or three times. Set aside.
4. Fill a medium pot with water and bring to boil. Take off heat. Add sun-dried tomatoes and Swiss chard. Let sit in water for 30 seconds. Drain and set aside.
5. After dough has risen, poke holes in it with a fork. Brush with rosemary-garlic oil. Bake in the oven for 12 to 14 minutes, until bread begins to brown. Remove from the oven. While slightly warm, spread crust evenly with hummus, and sprinkle with cooked sun-dried tomatoes and Swiss chard and red onion. Cut into 12 pieces.

DEFINITION

Hummus is a Middle Eastern dip or spread made from cooked chickpeas, sesame paste known as tahini, lemon juice, olive oil, and a few other spices. It is readily available, commercially made, and many flavored varieties are available.

TLC Tapenade Pizza with Caramelized Onions

The roasted red pepper and olive tapenade makes an excellent sauce for this whole-wheat pizza crust. Topped with *caramelized* onions, it's reminiscent of a classic French Provençal pizza.

Yield:	**Prep time:**	**Cook time:**	**Serving size:**
1 pizza (12 slices)	10 minutes	15 minutes	2 slices
Each serving has:			
240 calories	8 g fat	1 g saturated fat	0 mg cholesterol
5 g fiber	222 mg sodium		

1 tsp. corn or canola oil

1 lb. onions, thinly sliced

½ recipe Easy Whole-Wheat Pizza Dough (see recipe earlier in chapter) or 1 lb. pkg. frozen whole-wheat pizza dough, thawed

1 cup TLC Tapenade (see recipe in Chapter 17)

1. Heat the oven to 425°F.
2. Heat a medium saucepan over medium heat with 1 teaspoon corn oil, add onions, and sauté uncovered until caramelized about 15 minutes, stirring frequently. You can make the caramelized onions a day or two ahead and keep in the refrigerator.
3. While onions are cooking, roll out Easy Whole-Wheat Pizza Dough into a 12×12 square. Spread with TLC Tapenade and top with caramelized onions. Bake in the oven for 12 to 15 minutes or until crust is slightly brown.
4. Let cool for 5 minutes, cut into 12 pieces, and serve.

DEFINITION

When the natural sugars in onions are slowly heated, they turn a rich, dark brown color and produce a sweet, nutty flavor. This process is called **caramelization.**

Zucchini and Tomato Pizza

Impress your guests with this colorful, garlicky zucchini-and-tomato pizza sprinkled with Italian seasonings. It's perfect at the end of summer, when these vegetables are still in their prime.

Yield:	**Prep time:**	**Cook time:**	**Serving size:**
1 pizza (12 slices)	15 minutes	20 minutes	2 slices
Each serving has:			
176 calories	6 g fat	1 g saturated fat	0 mg cholesterol
3 g fiber	209 mg sodium		

½ recipe Easy Whole-Wheat Pizza Dough (see recipe earlier in chapter) or 1-lb. pkg. frozen whole-wheat pizza dough, thawed

2 tsp. olive oil

2 tsp. Spicy Italian Seasoning Blend (see recipe in Chapter 17) *or* 1 tsp. finely chopped fresh oregano and 1 tsp finely chopped fresh basil

1 garlic clove, crushed

1 medium zucchini, thinly sliced

2 medium tomatoes, thinly sliced

2 tsp. Parmesan cheese

½ tsp. freshly ground black pepper

1. Heat the oven to 425°F.
2. Roll out Easy Whole-Wheat Pizza Dough in a 12×12 square, and place on a pizza stone or cookie sheet sprayed with cooking spray. Let rise for about 15 minutes.
3. Mix olive oil with Spicy Italian Seasoning Blend and garlic. Heat in the microwave for 30 seconds, to allow flavors to blend. Brush evenly on Easy Whole-Wheat Pizza Dough.
4. Layer zucchini and tomato slices, alternating each and overlapping slightly to cover pizza. Sprinkle with Parmesan cheese and black pepper. Bake in the oven for 18 to 20 minutes.
5. Cut into 12 pieces and serve.

GOTCHA!

When it comes to fat, calories, and sodium, pizza is one of the worst offenders in the fast-food world. One slice of cheese pizza contains on average 240 calories, 10 grams total fat, 4.5 grams saturated fat, and some 530 milligrams sodium.

Beet and Orange Salad

Roasted thyme-scented beets and sweet oranges are dressed with a citrusy salad dressing in this hearty green salad. Sunflower seeds give crunch and extra protein.

Yield:	**Prep time:**	**Cook time:**	**Serving size:**
16 cups	25 minutes	30 minutes	4 cups
Each serving has:			
208 calories	8 g fat	1 g saturated fat	0 mg cholesterol
8 g fiber	443 mg sodium		

1 lb. beets, peeled and cut into $^1/_2$-in. dice
5 tsp. corn or vegetable oil, divided
1 tsp. fresh thyme leaves, minced
$^1/_4$ tsp. freshly ground black pepper
4 TB. orange juice
4 tsp. apple cider vinegar
2 TB. honey
2 tsp. Dijon mustard
$^1/_2$ tsp. sea salt or table salt
2 tsp. orange zest
12 cups mixed salad greens
2 oranges, sectioned
4 tsp. sunflower seeds

1. Heat the oven to 400°F.
2. Place beets in a medium roasting pan, and toss with 1 teaspoon corn oil, thyme, and $^1/_8$ teaspoon black pepper. Roast in the oven for 30 minutes or until beets are tender. Remove from the oven and set aside to cool.
3. While beets are cooking, in a small bowl, whisk together orange juice, apple cider vinegar, remaining 4 teaspoons corn oil, honey, Dijon mustard, sea salt, orange zest, and remaining $^1/_8$ teaspoon black pepper. Set aside dressing.
4. To assemble for each serving, place on a plate 3 cups salad greens and top with $^1/_2$ cup beets, $^1/_2$ orange sectioned, 1 teaspoon sunflower seeds, and 2 tablespoons dressing.

HEART-SMART HABITS

What's the best way to cook beets without staining your hands? Wear a pair of latex gloves. Another option is to peel and cut the beets under fast-running cold water.

Mediterranean Chickpea Salad

Bulgur wheat and chickpeas are the main ingredients in this vibrant salad pumped up with high-fiber green peas and red pepper. It tastes even better the next day.

Yield:	**Prep time:**	**Serving size:**	
6 cups	45 minutes	1 cup	
Each serving has:			
184 calories	5 g fat	1.3 g saturated fat	3 mg cholesterol
8 g fiber	266 mg sodium		

½ cup bulgur wheat (#1 fine grind; see sidebar)

1¼ cups boiling water

1 (15.5-oz.) can low-sodium chickpeas, drained and rinsed (or 1½ cups cooked)

6 oz. (about 1¼ cups) frozen peas, thawed

1 cup chopped green onions (green and white part), about 1 bunch

1 medium roasted red pepper, fresh or from a jar (about 5 oz.), ¼-in. dice

¼ cup chopped fresh oregano

Juice and zest of 1 lemon

1 TB. olive oil

¼ tsp. sea salt

¼ tsp. freshly ground black pepper

2 oz. low-fat feta, crumbled

1. Place bulgur wheat in a medium bowl and pour boiling water over it. Cover with plastic wrap and let sit for 20 to 30 minutes until liquid is absorbed and bulgur is fluffy and soft.
2. In another large bowl, gently mix low-sodium chickpeas, peas, green onions, roasted red pepper, oregano, lemon juice and zest, and olive oil. Fold in bulgur. Add sea salt, black pepper, and crumbled low-fat feta. Serve at room temperature or chilled.

DEFINITION

Bulgur is a whole wheat that is first steamed or parboiled, dried, and then crushed or ground. A staple in the Middle East, it is available in #1 fine, #2 medium, or #3 coarse grinds. One cup of bulgur has fewer calories, less fat, and more than twice the fiber of 1 cup of brown rice.

Tuna and Apple Salad

Canned tuna, apples, and walnuts take on a new twist when tossed with sliced fennel, mixed greens, and a tangy yogurt dressing. This salad is ideal for a light summer meal.

Yield:	**Prep time:**	**Serving size:**	
12 cups	5 minutes	3 cups	
Each serving has:			
242 calories	11 g fat	1.3 g saturated fat	11 mg cholesterol
4 g fiber	456 mg sodium		

- 1/2 cup nonfat plain Greek-style yogurt
- 4 TB. apple cider or apple juice
- 4 tsp. apple cider vinegar
- 4 tsp. olive oil
- 2 TB. honey
- 2 tsp. whole-grain mustard
- 1/2 tsp. kosher salt
- 1/4 tsp. freshly ground black pepper
- 8 cups mixed salad greens
- 2 cups chopped apples, unpeeled
- 1 (5-oz.) can or pouch tuna, drained
- 1 cup thinly sliced fennel
- 4 TB. chopped walnuts

1. In a small bowl, whisk together nonfat Greek-style yogurt, apple cider, apple cider vinegar, olive oil, honey, whole-grain mustard, kosher salt, and black pepper until well blended. Set aside.
2. In another large bowl, mix salad greens, apples, tuna, fennel, and walnuts. Pour dressing over top and gently toss together. Divide evenly among four plates and serve.

HEALTHFUL LIVING

What's the difference between white tuna and light tuna? White tuna is albacore tuna. It has a mild taste and is higher in omega-3 fatty acids, as well as the pollutant mercury. Light tuna, on the other hand, is from skipjack or yellowfin tuna. It is fishier tasting, is usually less expensive, and is lower in both omega-3 and mercury. The FDA recommends eating no more than 6 ounces of albacore tuna a week.

Curried Chicken Salad

This salad is more like a fruit salad with chicken than a chicken salad with fruit. Sweet apples and pineapple give a boost of vitamin C and fiber, while a sprinkle of almonds supplies the crunch. Make extra because this will disappear fast.

Yield:	**Prep time:**	**Serving size:**	
5 cups	20 minutes	1¼ cups	
Each serving has:			
86 calories	1.3 g fat	.2 g saturated fat	16 mg cholesterol
2 g fiber	69 mg sodium		

1 boneless, skinless chicken breast (about 4 oz.)

1 medium apple, cored and chopped, not peeled (about 1 cup)

½ cup pineapple chunks, cut into bite-size pieces

¼ cup nonfat plain Greek-style yogurt

½ tsp. *curry powder*

4 tsp. chopped red onion

¼ cup chopped celery

2 tsp. chopped almonds

Pinch sea salt (optional)

2 cups mixed salad greens

1. Place about 2 cups water in a medium saucepan and bring to a low simmer; bubbles will just begin breaking the top slowly. Add chicken breast. There should be enough water to cover. Cook on a low simmer for about 4 minutes or longer, depending on how thick your chicken breast is. Chicken should reach an internal temperature of 165°F. Remove chicken from water and let rest for 5 to 10 minutes.
2. While chicken is resting, in a large bowl, put apple, pineapple, nonfat Greek-style yogurt, curry powder, red onion, celery, and almonds. Cut chicken into bite-size pieces. Add to vegetable mixture and gently toss together until everything is incorporated. Add sea salt (if using). Serve on a bed of mixed salad greens.

DEFINITION

Curry powder is a blend of spices usually including cumin, coriander, red chiles, turmeric, and fenugreek. The mixture varies in strength and can be purchased mild or hot.

Arugula Tomato Salad with Red Pepper Tofu

Seasoned tofu takes the place of feta in this simple, eye-appealing arugula and tomato salad. For a more substantial meal, pair this slightly peppery salad with a soup or half sandwich.

Yield:	**Prep time:**	**Serving size:**	
10 cups	5 minutes	$2\frac{1}{2}$ cups	
Each serving has:			
78 calories	5 g fat	1 g saturated fat	0 mg cholesterol
2 g fiber	63 mg sodium		

- 8 cups arugula, roughly chopped
- 2 medium tomatoes, sliced into wedges
- $\frac{1}{2}$ cup Red Pepper Tofu (recipe in Chapter 17)
- 4 tsp. canola or vegetable oil
- $\frac{1}{4}$ tsp. freshly ground black pepper

1. In a large bowl, place arugula. Top with tomato wedges and sprinkle with Red Pepper Tofu. Drizzle with canola oil and sprinkle with black pepper. Toss together.
2. Divide evenly among four plates and serve.

Variation: If you don't have Red Pepper Tofu on hand, mix $\frac{1}{2}$ cup crumbled pressed tofu with 1 tablespoon apple cider vinegar, and sprinkle with $\frac{1}{8}$ teaspoon each dried basil and dried oregano and a dash of lemon juice. Toss together.

Watermelon Feta Salad

This salad is the perfect balance of sweet and salty. Lime adds a touch of tartness and basil adds an herbaceous note. It's ideal for the hot summer months when you don't feel like cooking. You can easily double this recipe.

Yield:	**Prep time:**	**Serving size:**	
2 cups watermelon mixture and 4 cups greens	10 minutes	1 cup watermelon mixture and 2 cups greens	
Each serving has:			
127 calories	7 g fat	1.6 g saturated fat	4 mg cholesterol
2 g fiber	215 mg sodium		

2 cups seedless watermelon, cut into bite-size pieces
1 oz. low-fat feta cheese, crumbled
2 TB. shredded fresh basil leaves
2 tsp. corn or grapeseed oil
2 tsp. lime juice
4 cups mixed salad greens

1. In a large bowl, toss watermelon and low-fat feta cheese.
2. In a small bowl, mix basil, corn oil, and lime juice. Pour basil mixture over watermelon and toss with mixed salad greens.
3. Divide evenly between two plates and serve.

Variation: For a lively twist, try replacing the oil and lime juice with 1 tablespoon of Orange-Lime Salad Dressing (recipe variation in Chapter 17).

HEALTHFUL LIVING

Watermelon is a rich source of lycopene (a red pigment), containing about 40 percent more lycopene than a raw tomato. In studies, lycopene has been shown to protect against heart disease, osteoporosis, and cancer.

Chapter 19

Fast and Easy

In This Chapter

- Simple sautés and stir-fries
- Mixed meals that come together in minutes
- Quick sandwiches, salads, and pastas

In this fast-paced world, few people have the time or inclination to spend long periods of time in the kitchen, particularly during the weekdays, when many people are busy. Instead, they grab fast, easy-to-make meals, sacrificing good nutrition and often taste, and jeopardizing their health and their heart along the way.

Just because you're on the TLC diet doesn't mean you'll be spending hours in the kitchen. In this chapter, I show you how to make healthful, flavorful meals in 40 minutes or less, while still including heart-smart vegetables and quick-cooking whole grains.

Eating well and eating healthfully does require more planning than just preparing a convenience food dinner or stopping at your local fast-food restaurant. But it's easy to plan healthful meals and have a set of fast-and-easy go-to recipes when your fridge and pantry are well stocked with good-for-you, low-calorie foods.

Remember, too, that cooking is a skill. The more you do it, the more accomplished you'll become. Consequently, chopping and cutting will get easier and faster with time. Consider some of these simple secrets to eating healthfully fast:

- Prepare grains that take under 20 minutes to cook, like couscous, quinoa, quick-cooking barley, and oatmeal.

- Sauté vegetables like onions, celery, zucchini, mushrooms, and peppers with different seasonings for an easy meal. If you're in a bind, you can buy them precut.
- Cut long-cooking vegetables in small pieces to shorten cooking time. You may even want to blanch them in boiling water for a few minutes first, to speed up cooking time. You can do this a day or two before. This works well for potatoes, sweet potatoes, green beans, carrots, broccoli, and cauliflower.
- Cut chicken, pork, or beef in small pieces to cook quickly.
- Cook a big batch of fresh dried beans when you have time, then store them in smaller containers in the fridge or freezer and pull them out when you need them. You can also use canned beans as long as you buy low-sodium brands and drain and rinse them before using.
- Have a variety of go-to spices or fresh herbs always ready so you can easily throw them in a dish to pump up flavor. Place them in small packages or ice cube trays in the freezer so you can enjoy fresh herbs all year.
- Keep a supply of fresh lemons and limes on hand to add a fast flavor boost to a meal.

Because most of the recipes in this chapter are centered around vegetables and grains, they typically contain some fiber, but if you want to punch up the fiber even more, I've included a Fiber Boost. Experiment with these recipes or use them as a guide to create your own. When you've mastered them, you'll realize just how fast and easy cooking the TLC way is—and along the way, you'll be surprised to find you've created your own quick go-to recipes without even trying!

Tilapia with Summer Squash

Simple and fresh characterizes this easy meal of sautéed tilapia paired with a colorful mélange of yellow squash, onions, and tomatoes, finished with capers, Italian parsley, and a splash of white wine.

Yield:	**Prep time:**	**Cook time:**	**Serving size:**
4 tilapia fillets and 4 cups vegetables	10 minutes	10 minutes	1 tilapia fillet and 1 cup vegetables
Each serving has:			
162 calories	4 g fat	1 g saturated fat	42 mg cholesterol
3 g fiber	109 mg sodium		

2 tsp. corn or olive oil

4 (3-oz.) boneless, skinless tilapia fillets

2 medium yellow squash or zucchini, sliced in ¼-in. rounds, then in half again (half-moon shapes)

¼ cup chopped red onion

1 garlic clove, minced

2 medium tomatoes, chopped

2 tsp. capers, chopped

1 cup Italian parsley, loosely packed, then chopped

½ cup white wine

¼ tsp. crushed red pepper flakes (optional)

1. In a medium sauté pan over medium-high heat, heat corn oil. Add tilapia fillets and sauté about 1 to 2 minutes on each side. Remove fillets from the pan and set aside.
2. In the same pan, add yellow squash, red onion, and garlic. Sauté for 2 minutes until slightly brown and zucchini has softened. Add tomatoes, capers, and Italian parsley. Cook for another 2 minutes. Pour in white wine, sprinkle in red pepper flakes (if using), and sauté for 1 minute so flavors blend. Return tilapia to the pan and reheat. Serve immediately.

HEALTHFUL LIVING

With only about 110 calories and 3 grams of fat (only 1 of them saturated), tilapia is a lean fish with a firm white flesh and mild taste. It's native to the Middle East and Africa, so only farm-raised tilapia is available in the United States. You'll find it in the fish section of the grocery store.

Citrus Salmon with Whole-Wheat Couscous

Citrus zest adds a jolt of flavor without adding fat, sugar, or salt. Here salmon is broiled with lime, lemon, and orange zest and then paired with orange-scented Israeli *couscous* and tangy arugula.

Yield:	**Prep time:**	**Cook time:**	**Serving size:**
4 salmon fillets with 4 cups couscous and arugula	10 minutes	15 minutes	1 salmon fillet with 1 cup couscous and arugula
Each serving has:			
328 calories	8 g fat	1 g saturated fat	52 mg cholesterol
5 g fiber	203 mg sodium		

Juice of $1\frac{1}{2}$ oranges

1 cup Israeli couscous

Freshly ground black pepper

8 cups roughly chopped arugula or spinach

1 tsp. lime zest

1 TB. orange zest

1 tsp. lemon zest

$\frac{1}{4}$ cup finely chopped white onion

$\frac{1}{4}$ cup finely chopped red pepper

4 (3-oz.) boneless, skinless salmon fillets

Juice of $\frac{1}{2}$ lime

2 TB. chopped cilantro

Salt to taste (optional)

1. Preheat the oven to 450°F.
2. Place juice of 1 orange in a 2-cup measure. Add enough water to make 2 cups. Heat orange juice–water mixture in a saucepot over medium-high heat until boiling. Add Israeli couscous and pinch of black pepper, and cook, covered, for about 8 to 10 minutes, until couscous is tender. Quickly stir in arugula and cover. Set aside for 10 minutes.
3. In another small bowl, stir together lime zest, orange zest, lemon zest, white onion, red pepper, and remaining juice of $\frac{1}{2}$ orange. Place salmon fillets in a $1\frac{1}{2}$-quart baking dish. Pour zest mixture over top of salmon. Bake in the oven for 10 minutes until fish is done and flakes easily from a fork. Set aside.

4. Mix couscous and arugula mixture with lime juice, cilantro, and salt (if using). Serve couscous and arugula mixture with salmon.

DEFINITION

Couscous is a small wheat pasta that is available in two sizes. Moroccan couscous (traditional couscous), has tiny grains and cooks in 5 minutes; Israeli couscous has larger round balls, is toasted, and cooks in about 8 to 10 minutes.

Tuna Fillet, Potato, and Green Bean Salad

Potatoes, tomatoes, and green beans are perfect complements to pan-seared tuna, which is drizzled with olive oil and lemon zest in this warm salad. This easy weeknight dinner can easily double as lunch the next day.

Yield:	**Prep time:**	**Cook time:**	**Serving size:**
7 cups	10 minutes	15 minutes	$1\frac{3}{4}$ cups
Each serving has:			
193 calories	8 g fat	1 g saturated fat	19 mg cholesterol
4 g fiber	167 mg sodium		

1 (6-oz.) tuna fillet

$\frac{1}{4}$ tsp. sea salt

$\frac{1}{4}$ tsp. freshly ground black pepper

$\frac{1}{2}$ lb. new or red bliss potatoes, cut into $\frac{1}{2}$-in. pieces

$\frac{1}{2}$ lb. green beans, cleaned and trimmed, cut in 1-in. pieces

2 medium tomatoes, cut in bite-size wedges

2 tsp. lemon zest

2 tsp. fresh chopped oregano

2 tsp. fresh basil

6 tsp. olive oil

2 clove garlic, minced

4 TB. red onion, diced

1. Heat a small sauté pan over high heat. Spray with cooking spray and add tuna fillet. Sear tuna, cooking 2 to 3 minutes on each side. Sprinkle with $\frac{1}{8}$ teaspoon sea salt and $\frac{1}{8}$ teaspoon black pepper. Set aside.
2. In a 3-quart pot, bring 4 cups water to a boil. Reduce heat to a slow boil and drop in new potatoes. Cook about 6 minutes or until tender. Drain and rinse potatoes under cool water, and set aside.
3. In the same 3-quart pot, bring 3 cups water to a boil. Reduce heat to a slow boil and add green beans. Cook $2\frac{1}{2}$ minutes, then drain and rinse under cool water.
4. In a large bowl, toss potatoes, green beans, tomatoes, tuna, lemon zest, oregano, basil, olive oil, garlic, and red onion. Sprinkle with remaining $\frac{1}{8}$ teaspoon salt and remaining $\frac{1}{8}$ teaspoon black pepper. Serve on a bed of lettuce or alone.

HEALTHFUL LIVING

Although potatoes have gotten a reputation for being "fattening," the truth is, one medium naked baked potato has only 110 calories. Plus, it provides a good amount of vitamin C, potassium, vitamin B_6, fiber, and iron. Just don't fry it!

Maple-Glazed Scallops with Sautéed Spinach

In this light dish, seared scallops are dressed with sweet maple syrup, lemon, and thyme and served on top of a bed of sautéed spinach and kale. To finish off the dish, pair it with a nutty wild rice blend.

Yield:	**Prep time:**	**Cook time:**	**Serving size:**
8 scallops and 4 cups greens	15 minutes	20 minutes	2 scallops and 1 cup greens
Each serving has:			
169 calories	4 g fat	.3 g saturated fat	28 mg cholesterol
2 g fiber	388 mg sodium		

1 TB. lemon juice
1 TB. maple syrup
1 tsp. fresh thyme leaves
2 tsp. Dijon mustard
$\frac{1}{4}$ tsp. red pepper flakes
2 tsp. corn or vegetable oil
$\frac{1}{4}$ cup chopped onion
1 clove garlic, minced
4 cups chopped kale
4 cups chopped spinach
$\frac{1}{4}$ cup water
12 oz. large or jumbo scallops (about 8)
$\frac{1}{4}$ cup white wine
$\frac{1}{4}$ tsp. sea salt or table salt
Freshly ground black pepper

1. In a small bowl, whisk lemon juice, maple syrup, thyme, Dijon mustard, and red pepper flakes. Set aside.
2. Heat 1 teaspoon corn oil in a medium sauté pan over medium-high heat. Add onion, garlic, and kale. Cook for 5 minutes until onion begins to soften, then cover and cook for another 5 minutes.
3. Add spinach and water. Cover and cook 5 minutes more until greens are wilted. Place in a serving bowl and keep warm.
4. In another medium saucepan, heat remaining 1 teaspoon corn oil over medium-high heat. Add scallops to pan and cook 2 minutes on each side until edges are brown. Pour in sauce and cook for 20 to 30 seconds. Pour in white wine. Cook for another 10 seconds, then remove from heat. Sprinkle with sea salt and black pepper.

5. Pour scallops and sauce over top of greens and serve immediately.

HEALTHFUL LIVING

Of all the leafy greens, kale is considered king. A nutritional superfood, 1 cup raw kale provides more than 200 percent of the daily value for vitamin A, more than 130 percent of vitamin C, and a whopping 680 percent of vitamin K.

Sicilian Sardine Pasta

This Sicilian-inspired recipe features sardines in a caper-lemon-parsley-tomato sauce served over whole-wheat pasta. Lightly browned breadcrumbs are sprinkled over top in place of cheese.

Yield:	**Prep time:**	**Cook time:**	**Serving size:**
7 cups	10 minutes	25 minutes	1¾ cups
Each serving has:			
353 calories	8 g fat	1 g saturated fat	4 mg cholesterol
7 g fiber	240 mg sodium		

8 oz. whole-wheat penne pasta

3 oz. whole-wheat bread, chopped, crust removed

2 tsp. olive oil

1 small onion, diced

1 (3.75-oz.) can boneless, skinless sardines in olive oil

1 medium tomato, diced

1 TB. capers, roughly chopped

½ cup Italian parsley, roughly chopped

1 tsp. lemon zest

1 TB. shredded basil

1. Fill a 1½-quart pot with water and bring to boil. Add whole-wheat penne pasta and cook for 12 minutes. Drain, reserving 1 cup pasta water.
2. Place whole-wheat bread in a food processor and chop about 15 seconds or until bread is in about ¼-inch pieces. In a large saucepan, sauté breadcrumbs in olive oil until lightly browned, about 3 to 4 minutes. Take out of the pan and set aside.
3. In the same pan, sauté onion until lightly browned, about 3 to 4 minutes. Add sardines in olive oil, tomato, pasta, and capers. Cook about 2 minutes.
4. Add ½ cup reserved pasta water, Italian parsley, lemon zest, basil, and breadcrumbs, and sauté another 30 seconds. (Add remaining pasta water if it seems dry.) Serve immediately.

HEALTHFUL LIVING

A small silvery fish rich in omega-3 fatty acids, vitamin B_{12}, selenium, and vitamin D (if you eat the small soft bones), sardines are most popular around the Mediterranean region but are also found in the Atlantic and Pacific oceans.

Chicken with Lemon-Barley Pilaf and Broccoli

This colorful, nontraditional *pilaf* is as beautiful as it is good for you. Broccoli, carrots, and raisins are tossed together with chewy barley and tender bite-size pieces of chicken.

Yield:	**Prep time:**	**Cook time:**	**Serving size:**
5 cups	10 minutes	25 minutes	$1\frac{1}{4}$ cups
Each serving has:			
291 calories	4 g fat	.4 g saturated fat	32 mg cholesterol
7 g fiber	190 mg sodium		

- $\frac{1}{2}$ cup raisins
- 3 cups water
- 2 tsp. corn oil or vegetable oil
- 8 oz. chicken breast, cut into 1-in. pieces
- 1 medium onion, chopped into 1-in. pieces (about 1 cup)
- 1 medium carrot, peeled and julienned into 1-in. strips
- 1 cup quick-cooking barley
- $\frac{1}{2}$ tsp. ground caraway seed, ground from seed with coffee grinder
- $\frac{1}{2}$ tsp. ground ginger
- $\frac{1}{2}$ tsp. grated lemon zest
- 1 cup cooked broccoli florets (or thawed from frozen), cut into 1-in. pieces
- $\frac{1}{4}$ tsp. kosher salt

1. In a small bowl, soak raisins in 1 cup water for about 15 minutes. While raisins are soaking, heat 1 teaspoon corn oil in a medium saucepan. Add chicken and sauté about 4 or 5 minutes. Remove chicken, tent with foil, and set aside to keep warm.
2. To the same saucepan you cooked chicken in, add remaining 1 teaspoon oil, onion, and carrot. Cook over medium-high heat for about 5 minutes or until soft. Stir in quick-cooking barley, caraway seed, and ginger, and cook 2 more minutes, stirring frequently. Pour in remaining 2 cups water. Cover, cook, and simmer for 10 minutes.

3. When mixture is almost cooked, place raisins, chicken, lemon zest, and broccoli on top of barley. Sprinkle with kosher salt and do not stir. Cover and cook for 5 minutes. Uncover, stir, and serve.

DEFINITION

Pilaf originated in the Middle East but is the standard way to cook whole grains in many Mediterranean and Latin countries, too. In a pilaf, the grain is sautéed or browned in butter or oil with vegetables for a few minutes before the liquid is added.

Turkey Sloppy Joes

This more healthful version of a sloppy joe keeps the sweet, tangy sauce but uses ground turkey in place of ground beef. Mashed kidney beans give it a heftier texture. You won't even notice the difference.

Yield:	**Prep time:**	**Cook time:**	**Serving size:**
4 cup	10 minutes	20 minutes	1 cup
Each serving has:			
240 calories	6 g fat	1.5 g saturated fat	44 mg cholesterol
7 g fiber	319 mg sodium		

1 tsp. corn or canola oil

8 oz. lean ground turkey

1 small onion, finely diced

½ medium green bell pepper, finely diced

1 medium stalk celery, finely diced

1 garlic clove, minced

2 tsp. balsamic vinegar

1 tsp. Worcestershire sauce

¼ cup ketchup

1 cup crushed tomatoes

1 TB. brown sugar

⅛ tsp. freshly ground black pepper

½ tsp finely chopped fresh thyme

½ tsp. dry mustard

1½ cups water

1½ cups cooked red kidney beans

1. In a 2-quart saucepot, heat corn oil over medium-high heat. Brown turkey in oil, stirring to break up, about 4 minutes. Add onion, green bell pepper, celery, and garlic. Cook another 3 or 4 minutes until vegetables begin to soften.
2. Add balsamic vinegar, Worcestershire sauce, ketchup, tomatoes, brown sugar, black pepper, thyme, dry mustard, water, and red kidney beans. Stir to incorporate. Mash beans with a potato masher to incorporate into meat mixture. Simmer 10 minutes.
3. Serve alone with rice or on buns or bread as a sandwich.

Fiber Boost: Serve on 1 cup of cooked quinoa to boost fiber another 5 grams.

HEALTHFUL LIVING

The original sloppy joe was created in the 1920s by an Iowa restaurateur who mixed sweet tomato sauce (ketchup) and seasoning with ground beef and placed it between two slices of bread.

Cuban Pork with Black Beans and Sweet Potatoes

Pork tenderloin, sweet potatoes, and black beans are the main components of this South American–inspired stew. Using canned or precooked black beans and small diced sweet potatoes makes this meal cook in a flash.

Yield: 6 cups	**Prep time:** 15 minutes	**Cook time:** 20 minutes	**Serving size:** $1\frac{1}{2}$ cups
Each serving has:			
316 calories	4 g fat	1 g saturated fat	36 mg cholesterol
11 g fiber	341 mg sodium		

- 2 tsp. corn or canola oil
- 8 oz. lean pork tenderloin or loin, cut into $\frac{1}{2}$-in. pieces
- 1 medium onion, chopped
- 3 garlic cloves, minced
- 3 TB. all-purpose or whole-wheat flour
- 2 cups water
- 1 lb. sweet potato, peeled and cut into $\frac{1}{2}$-in. pieces
- 1 TB. fresh oregano, finely chopped
- 1 tsp. ground cumin
- $\frac{1}{8}$ tsp. freshly ground black pepper
- $\frac{1}{2}$ tsp. kosher salt
- $1\frac{3}{4}$ cup cooked black beans
- 1 tsp. hot sauce
- $\frac{1}{2}$ cup loosely packed cilantro, roughly chopped

1. Heat corn oil over medium-high heat in a large saucepan. Add pork tenderloin and brown, stirring frequently, about 3 minutes. Mix in onion and garlic. Cook 2 more minutes. Stir in all-purpose flour, mixing constantly until flour is moistened, about 1 minute.
2. Pour in water, scraping up brown bits from the bottom. Bring to a boil and cook about 2 minutes. Add sweet potato, oregano, cumin, black pepper, and kosher salt. Reduce to a simmer, cover, and cook 10 minutes.
3. When sweet potato is soft, add black beans and simmer 5 more minutes. Take off heat and finish with hot sauce and cilantro. Serve immediately plain or over rice.

HEALTHFUL LIVING

Sweet potatoes are brimming with vitamin A. One medium baked sweet potato contains more than four times the recommended daily intake for this nutrient. Sweet potatoes are also high in fiber, vitamin C, potassium, and manganese.

Beef with Soba Noodles and Vegetables

Soba noodles are commonly eaten in Japanese cuisine. Here they are combined with stir-fried steak and crunchy vegetables in an Asian-style noodle salad that can be served warm or cold.

Yield:	**Prep time:**	**Cook time:**	**Serving size:**
8 cups	20 minutes	7 minutes	2 cups
Each serving has:			
240 calories	7 g fat	1.5 g saturated fat	21 mg cholesterol
4 g fiber	165 mg sodium		

2 tsp. sesame seed oil

6 oz. sirloin steak, very thinly sliced

2 oz. plus 1/4 cup water

7 oz. soba noodles

1/2 cup green onions, chopped

1 garlic clove, minced

1 cup edamame, cooked per pkg. directions

2 cups cabbage, finely shredded

1/2 cup red bell pepper, diced

4 tsp. low-sodium soy sauce

2 tsp. sesame seeds

2 tsp. honey

1/2 tsp. hot sauce

1. Heat sesame seed oil in a seasoned wok or sauté pan over high heat. Sear sirloin steak in the wok about 1 minute on each side. Remove from the wok and set aside.
2. Add 2 ounces water to the hot wok and scrape up brown bits. Pour liquid into cup measure and set aside.
3. Bring a pot of water to a boil over high heat, reduce to a low boil, and add soba noodles. Cook 4 to 5 minutes, then rinse under cold water and set aside.
4. In a large bowl, toss noodles with steak, green onions, garlic, edamame, cabbage, and red bell pepper.
5. In a small bowl, whisk together low-sodium soy sauce, 1 teaspoon sesame seeds, honey, hot sauce, and remaining 1/4 cup water. Pour over noodles. Then gently toss together. To serve, sprinkle remaining 1 teaspoon sesame seeds on top.

DEFINITION

Brown **soba noodles** (also called buckwheat noodles) are made from buckwheat flour and have a strong nutty flavor. They are prepared with a number of different meat, fish, poultry, and vegetable dishes and can be served hot or cold.

TLC Steak Fajitas

Extra vegetables pump up this traditional fajita chock-full of peppers, tomatoes, onions, and mushrooms. Wrapped in a large flour tortilla, it makes a hearty and filling meal.

Yield:	**Prep time:**	**Cook time:**	**Serving size:**
4 fajitas	10 minutes	8 minutes	1 fajita
Each serving has:			
481 calories	12 g fat	3 g saturated fat	50 cholesterol
8 g fiber	486 mg sodium		

8 oz. top round steak, thinly sliced in 2-in.-long strips

2 TB. fajita seasoning blend

2 tsp. corn or canola oil

4 oz. red bell pepper, thinly sliced

4 oz. green bell pepper, thinly sliced

4 oz. yellow bell pepper, thinly sliced

1 medium onion, thinly sliced

4 oz. mushrooms, sliced

1 large tomato, cut in wedges

4 (10-in.) flour tortillas

Nonfat plain Greek-style yogurt for garnish

1. Rub top round steak with fajita seasoning blend and set aside.
2. Heat corn oil in a large sauté pan over high heat. Add steak and sauté meat for 2 minutes on each side.
3. Add red bell pepper, green bell pepper, yellow bell pepper, and onion, stirring frequently. Cover and cook for 3 minutes on medium-high heat.
4. Add mushrooms and tomato to the pan. Cook 2 more minutes, covered. To serve, place 1¼ cups fajita mixture in center of flour tortilla, fold over center, and wrap up each side. Top with a dollop of nonfat Greek-style yogurt.

HEART-SMART HABITS

Be sure to choose a fajita spice blend with no salt or sugar added.

Spicy Hummus in a Pita

Why buy commercial hummus when all it takes is a few minutes to whip up a batch of your own? Served on a pita with lettuce, tomato, and cucumber, it makes a quick and easy dinner.

Yield:	Prep time:	Serving size:	
8 pitas with 2 cups hummus	10 minutes	1 pita with $\frac{1}{4}$ cup hummus	
Each serving has:			
179 calories	6 g fat	1 g saturated fat	0 mg cholesterol
6 g fiber	204 mg sodium		

- $1\frac{1}{4}$ cups cooked chickpeas (if using canned, drain and rinse)
- 1 dried ancho pepper, seeded and stem removed, cut into pieces
- $\frac{1}{4}$ cup tahini (sesame seed paste)
- $\frac{1}{4}$ cup water
- 2 TB. chopped green onion
- $\frac{1}{4}$ tsp. cumin
- Juice of $\frac{1}{2}$ lemon
- 2 garlic cloves
- $\frac{1}{8}$ tsp. sea salt
- $\frac{1}{8}$ tsp. freshly ground black pepper
- 4 whole-wheat pitas
- 4 cups shredded lettuce
- 2 cups chopped tomato
- 2 cups chopped cucumber, seeded and peeled

1. Place chickpeas, ancho pepper, tahini, water, green onion, cumin, lemon juice, garlic, sea salt, and black pepper in a food processor. Purée for 30 seconds, stop, and scrape down the bowl. Repeat two more times.
2. To assemble, place $\frac{1}{4}$ cup hummus in a whole-wheat pita and top with $\frac{1}{2}$ cup shredded lettuce, $\frac{1}{4}$ cup chopped tomato, and $\frac{1}{4}$ cup chopped cucumber.

Variation: Hummus is extremely versatile. Change the flavor by adding roasted red pepper, black olives, or sun-dried tomatoes; use cilantro, basil, or parsley in place of the green onion; or add different spices like chili powder or curry powder.

Vegetarian/Vegan

Chapter 20

In This Chapter

- Simply sensational plant food
- Amazing Asian-inspired tofu dishes
- Virtuous vegan cuisine

Although there are many types of vegetarians, in general most people classify this group as people who don't eat any meat, fish, or poultry, but who do eat eggs, cheese, and dairy products. Vegans are people who don't eat any meat, fish, poultry, eggs, or dairy products, like cheese or yogurt. Vegetarians and vegans who follow a sound, well-balanced, healthful diet have lower rates of all kinds of diseases, including heart disease, diabetes, and high blood pressure.

On the TLC diet, you'll be focusing more on plant-based foods and less on animal foods. Thus, you'll be eating several vegetarian and vegan meals a week. Eating vegetarian requires a bit more creativity, not to mention a whole lot more healthful foods. Variety is the key to a sound plant-based diet, and for that, you need a rainbow of color—think red, green, yellow, purple, and orange.

You've already seen some vegetarian and vegan recipes in previous chapters—consider Asparagus with Sun-Dried Tomatoes, Quinoa, and Basmati Rice (see Chapter 16); the salads and pizzas in Chapter 18; and Spicy Hummus in a Pita (see Chapter 19). Now it's time to dig in deeper with these vegetarian and vegan dishes inspired by cuisines from around the world.

I've divided these recipes into two sections, "Quick Recipes for When You're in a Hurry" and "Weekend Recipes for When You Have the Time." Designed to be versatile as well as tasty and TLC healthful, these meals will get you well on your way to including more plant-based foods in your diet. Feature them on weekends, on weekdays, and at parties. You and your family will love them.

Quick Recipes for When You're in a Hurry

These are meals you want to have when time is short or you don't know what to make. Keep staples like favorite vegetables, tofu, bread, and some cooked grains in the house, and you'll always have a meal at hand.

Grilled Eggplant and Tomato Panini

What could be easier than making a grilled eggplant-and-tomato sandwich? Use a panini maker to grill the vegetables as well as the sandwich, and you'll save even more time.

Yield:	**Prep time:**	**Cook time:**	**Serving size:**
2 sandwiches	10 minutes	10 minutes	1 sandwich
Each serving has:			
255 calories	9 g fat	1.5 g saturated fat	4 mg cholesterol
6 g fiber	463 mg sodium		

1 tsp. basil, finely chopped

1 small garlic clove, crushed

2 TB. low-fat canola mayonnaise

8 oz. eggplant, peeled and cut into 16 thin slices, $\frac{1}{8}$ in. thick

$\frac{1}{4}$ tsp. garlic powder

$\frac{1}{4}$ tsp. onion powder

$\frac{1}{8}$ tsp. ground black pepper

1 tsp. chopped fresh oregano

1 tsp. corn or olive oil

4 slices whole-wheat Italian bread

1 medium tomato, thinly sliced (about 8 slices)

$\frac{1}{2}$ oz. low-fat mozzarella cheese, shredded

1. In a small bowl, whisk together basil, garlic, and low-fat canola mayonnaise. Set aside.
2. Heat a panini maker or small sauté pan. In a medium bowl, sprinkle eggplant slices with garlic powder, onion powder, black pepper, and oregano, and drizzle with corn oil while tossing together until coated. Place eggplant on the panini maker and close, or place on a sauté pan and press down with cover. Grill for about 3 minutes. Set aside. You may need to do this in several batches, depending on how big your panini maker is.
3. Place whole-wheat Italian bread slices on a flat work surface. Spread each slice with 1 teaspoon basil-garlic mayonnaise. Top one slice with 4 slices of tomato, 8 slices of grilled eggplant, and half the low-fat mozzarella cheese. Cover with top. Repeat with the other slice of bread.

4. Spread remaining 2 teaspoons of garlic mayonnaise on outside of each sandwich, both sides ($\frac{1}{2}$ teaspoon on each side of bread). Place on panini maker or in a small hot sauté pan and grill 3 minutes or until cheese begins to melt and bread has browned.

HEART-SMART HABITS

Low-fat canola mayonnaise has half the calories of regular mayonnaise, plus no saturated fat or cholesterol, making it a good choice on the TLC diet. Olive oil mayonnaise, although lower in calories, fat, and saturated fat than regular mayonnaise, is higher in calories, fat, and saturated fat than canola mayonnaise.

Spicy Tofu and Green Bean Stir-Fry

Green beans and tofu are coated with a gingery soy sauce, then tossed with red pepper, sesame seeds, and garlic.

Yield:	**Prep time:**	**Cook time:**	**Serving size:**
4 cups	30 minutes	10 minutes	1 cup
Each serving has:			
114 calories	6 g fat	.7 g saturated fat	0 mg cholesterol
3 g fiber	226 mg sodium		

1 TB. low-sodium soy sauce

1 tsp. granulated sugar

¼ cup water

2 tsp. canola oil

7 oz. extra-firm tofu, pressed with paper towels to remove water

½ small onion, diced

2 garlic cloves, crushed

1 TB. fresh ginger, chopped

8 oz. green beans, trimmed and cut in half

½ sweet red bell pepper, diced

1 tsp. sesame seed oil

1 TB. sesame seeds

¼ tsp. dried red pepper flakes

1. In a small bowl, mix low-sodium soy sauce, sugar, and water. Set aside.
2. Heat canola oil in a wok or sauté pan over medium-high heat until hot. Stir-fry tofu until brown on all edges, about 3 to 4 minutes. Remove from the pan.
3. Stir-fry onion, garlic, and ginger until caramelized, about 1 to 2 minutes. Add green beans and sweet red bell pepper with sesame seed oil and stir-fry another 2 minutes. Be careful not to burn onions and garlic.
4. Pour in soy sauce mixture and reserved tofu, and sauté 1 minute. Sprinkle with sesame seeds and red pepper flakes. Toss and serve over brown rice, soba noodles, or whole-wheat pasta, or eat plain.

GOTCHA!

Asian condiments like soy sauce and oyster sauce are typically high in sodium, and many contain sugar in the form of high-fructose corn syrup. Choose a low-sodium option and use sparingly.

Cucumber Cashew Salad

Thailand meets India in this crunchy cucumber salad that pairs cucumber and carrot with cashews, lime juice, coconut flakes, and garam masala. This salad is great for hot summer days.

Yield:	Prep time:	Serving size:	
4 cups	15 minutes	1 cup	
Each serving has:			
136 calories	9 g fat	3 g saturated fat	0 mg cholesterol
3 g fiber	161 mg sodium		

- 2 medium cucumbers, peeled, seeded, and cut into $\frac{1}{2}$-in. dice
- $\frac{1}{4}$ cup small diced yellow bell pepper
- 1 small carrot, peeled, cut into $\frac{1}{4}$-in. dice
- $\frac{1}{4}$ cup cashew pieces, roasted
- 3 TB. large-flake unsweetened coconut
- 1 TB. lime juice
- 1 tsp. lime zest
- 1 tsp. granulated sugar
- 2 tsp. olive oil
- $\frac{1}{4}$ tsp. sea salt
- 2 TB. chopped green onions
- $\frac{1}{2}$ cup cilantro, chopped
- $\frac{1}{4}$ tsp. dried red pepper flakes
- 1 garlic clove, crushed
- $\frac{1}{8}$ tsp. ground cumin
- 1 tsp. garam masala

1. In a large bowl, mix cucumbers, yellow bell pepper, carrot, cashew pieces, unsweetened coconut, lime juice, lime zest, sugar, olive oil, sea salt, green onions, cilantro, red pepper flakes, garlic, cumin, and garam masala. Gently toss together to blend.
2. Serve at room temperature or chilled.

Variation: Substitute peanuts for the cashews, substitute Thai basil for the cilantro, and add 2 teaspoons rice vinegar.

Kale, Farro, and Fennel Salad

Cooking the farro a day ahead of time saves time and allows this salad to come together in minutes. Don't skip blanching the kale; not only does it make the leaves more tender, but it also gives this salad a burst of color and makes it last longer.

Yield:	**Prep time:**	**Cook time:**	**Serving size:**
9 cups	20 minutes	5 minutes	$1\frac{1}{2}$ cups
Each serving has:			
265 calories	12 g fat	2 g saturated fat	0 mg cholesterol
8 g fiber	132 mg sodium		

- $\frac{1}{2}$ bunch kale (about 8 oz.), cut into 1-in. pieces
- $1\frac{1}{4}$ cups cooked farro ($\frac{1}{2}$ cup raw)
- 1 cup peas, thawed from frozen or fresh cooked
- 1 cup sliced fennel
- $\frac{1}{2}$ cup red onion, thinly sliced
- 1 avocado, peeled and diced (about 8 oz.)
- 1 medium roasted red pepper
- $\frac{1}{4}$ cup roasted, salted pumpkin seeds
- $\frac{1}{2}$ cup green onion, roughly chopped
- Juice of $\frac{1}{2}$ lemon
- 1 TB. olive oil
- 1 cup parsley, loosely packed
- 2 tsp. honey
- $\frac{1}{2}$ cup nonfat plain Greek-style yogurt
- $\frac{1}{8}$ tsp. ground black pepper
- 2 tsp. apple cider vinegar
- 1 garlic clove, crushed

1. Fill a large stockpot with water and bring to a boil. Blanch kale in boiling water for 10 seconds. Remove with slotted spoon and immediately plunge in ice water bath for 10 to 15 seconds. Remove and dry on paper towels, or place in a salad spinner to remove moisture.
2. Place kale, farro, peas, fennel, red onion, avocado, red pepper, and pumpkin seeds in a large bowl and toss together.
3. Put green onion, lemon juice, olive oil, parsley, honey, nonfat Greek-style yogurt, black pepper, apple cider vinegar, and garlic in a food processor and blend for 2 minutes until smooth.
4. To serve, toss dressing with salad.

Summer Vegetable Pasta

This dish featuring the vegetables of summer couldn't be easier. Simply sauté zucchini, tomatoes, mushrooms, and artichokes, and toss with pasta and fresh herbs to make a light, colorful dish that's great for informal get-togethers.

Yield:	**Prep time:**	**Cook time:**	**Serving size:**
8 cups	10 minutes	20 minutes	2 cups
Each serving has:			
255 calories	7 g fat	1 g saturated fat	1 mg cholesterol
9 g fiber	203 mg sodium		

- 6 oz. rotelli or spiral pasta
- 4 tsp. olive oil
- 4 oz. zucchini, cut into ¼-in.-thick half-moons
- 4 oz. yellow squash, cut into ¼-in.-thick half-moons
- 1 medium tomato, diced
- 4 oz. mushrooms, sliced ¼ in. thick
- 6 oz. artichoke hearts thawed from frozen, cut in quarters
- ½ cup red onion, diced
- 2 garlic cloves, crushed
- ½ cup loosely packed basil, roughly chopped
- ¼ cup loosely packed fresh oregano, roughly chopped
- ¼ tsp. freshly ground black pepper
- ¼ tsp. sea salt
- 4 tsp. grated Parmesan cheese

1. Fill a 4-quart pot with 3 quarts water and bring to a boil. Add rotelli pasta and cook 12 minutes or until al dente. Drain and set aside.
2. Heat a large sauté pan over medium-high heat and add olive oil. When hot, add zucchini, yellow squash, tomato, mushrooms, artichoke hearts, red onion, and garlic to the pan. Sauté 4 to 5 minutes until soft, stirring frequently.
3. Mix in cooked pasta, basil, oregano, black pepper, and sea salt. Sauté 2 more minutes. Serve with 1 teaspoon Parmesan cheese per serving.

HEALTHFUL LIVING

Although considered a vegetable, squash is botanically a fruit. It was part of the "three sisters"—squash, beans, and corn—grown by Native Americans. There are two categories: summer squash, like zucchini and yellow squash, and winter squash, like pumpkin and butternut.

Couscous, Butternut Squash, and Green Beans

Whole-wheat couscous, butternut squash, green beans, and raisins make up this African-inspired dish, which is both sweet and spicy. It's topped with salty feta cheese to round out the flavors.

Yield:	**Prep time:**	**Cook time:**	**Serving size:**
6 cups	10 minutes	10 minutes	1 cup
Each serving has:			
194 calories	4 g fat	2 g saturated fat	10 mg cholesterol
6 g fiber	180 mg sodium		

1 tsp. corn or canola oil

$\frac{1}{2}$ cup red onion, finely diced

$1\frac{1}{2}$ cups butternut squash, cut into $\frac{1}{4}$-in. pieces

$\frac{1}{3}$ cup water

$1\frac{1}{2}$ cups green beans, cut into 1-in. pieces

$1\frac{2}{3}$ cup low-sodium vegetable broth

$\frac{1}{4}$ cup raisins

1 cup whole-wheat couscous

1 cup loosely packed Italian parsley, roughly chopped

$\frac{1}{4}$ tsp. cinnamon

$\frac{1}{2}$ tsp. ground cumin

$\frac{1}{8}$ tsp. ground black pepper

$\frac{1}{2}$ cup crumbled feta cheese

1. Heat corn oil in a 4-quart pot over medium-high heat. Sauté red onion and butternut squash for about 4 minutes until lightly browned. Add water and green beans. Simmer, covered, about 3 minutes.
2. Pour in low-sodium vegetable broth and bring to a boil. Mix in raisins, whole-wheat couscous, Italian parsley, cinnamon, cumin, and black pepper. Cover, take off the heat, and set aside for 5 minutes. Uncover and fluff with a fork. Sprinkle crumbled feta cheese and gently toss together. Serve immediately.

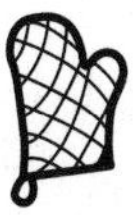

HEART-SMART HABITS

To have nice, plump raisins, place them in water, drain, and then put them back in their bag (they will still be slightly wet). Seal and store in the refrigerator. The raisins will absorb the water remaining on them and plump as they sit.

Grilled Tofu and Avocado Cream

Tofu takes on whatever flavors you pair it with. Here grilled tofu is seasoned with basil, garlic, and thyme and then topped with a light, creamy avocado-cucumber sauce flavored with just a hint of ginger.

Yield:	**Prep time:**	**Cook time:**	**Serving size:**
14 oz. tofu with 1 cup avocado cream	45 minutes	10 minutes	$3\frac{1}{2}$ oz. tofu with 2 tablespoons avocado cream
Each serving has:			
106 calories	6 g fat	1 g saturated fat	0 mg cholesterol
2 g fiber	92 mg sodium		

1 (14-oz.) pkg. firm or extra-firm tofu, cut in 8 slices

$\frac{1}{2}$ avocado

6 oz. English cucumber, peeled and seeded and roughly chopped

2 TB. unsweetened plain soy milk

2 TB. fresh parsley, roughly chopped

$\frac{1}{2}$ tsp. grated ginger

$\frac{1}{2}$ TB. rice wine vinegar

$\frac{1}{2}$ TB. chopped onion

$\frac{1}{4}$ tsp. chili sauce

Dash sea salt

1 TB. finely chopped fresh basil

$\frac{1}{4}$ tsp. freshly ground black pepper

1 tsp. garlic powder

1. Press water out of firm tofu by placing tofu pieces on a wire rack. Cover with several paper towels, and place heavy weight on top. Let tofu sit for 30 minutes, changing the paper towels frequently.
2. While tofu is pressing, make avocado cream. In a food processor, place avocado, English cucumber, unsweetened soy milk, parsley, ginger, rice wine vinegar, onion, chili sauce, and sea salt. Purée on high for about 40 seconds until smooth. Set aside.
3. Heat a griddle pan over medium-high heat. Sprinkle pressed tofu evenly with basil, $\frac{1}{2}$ of the black pepper, and garlic powder on each side. Spray tofu with cooking spray and grill for about 3 minutes on each side until browned.
4. To serve, place grilled tofu slices in bowls and top each with 2 tablespoons avocado cream. You will have about $\frac{1}{2}$ cup avocado cream left over; toss it with pasta, rice, or vegetables.

HEALTHFUL LIVING

Although more than 50 varieties of avocado exist, only two are commercially sold throughout the United States: the Hass avocado, from California, and the Florida avocado. The Hass avocado is small and bumpy, with dark purple skin; the Florida avocado is much bigger, with glossy green skin and less fat than the Hass.

Weekend Recipes for When You Have the Time

Make these meals when you have more time in the kitchen, like on a leisurely weekend. They are also good for potlucks and barbecues. Some, like the Vietnamese Salad Rolls, are more fun when you have a group of people to help you.

Vietnamese Salad Rolls

Fresh and healthful, these mini salad rolls have the peanut sauce right inside. Don't be afraid to change up the vegetables and herbs, depending on what you like. These are best made in big batches to enjoy with friends.

Yield:	**Prep time:**	**Cook time:**	**Serving size:**
24 rolls	50 minutes	7 minutes	2 rolls
Each serving has:			
207 calories	10 g fat	2 g saturated fat	0 mg cholesterol
3 g fiber	93 mg sodium		

- 1/4 cup unsalted, all-natural creamy peanut butter
- 1/2 tsp. sesame seed oil
- 1 tsp. low-sodium soy sauce
- 1/2 tsp. grated ginger
- 1/4 tsp. hot sauce
- 3 TB. hot water
- 1 TB. rice vinegar
- 1/2 tsp. sesame seeds
- 14 oz. extra-firm tofu, sliced into 1/4-in. slices
- 2 medium carrots, peeled and cut into 3-in. matchstick pieces
- 2 small cucumbers, peeled, seeded, and cut into 3-in. matchstick pieces
- 2 green onions, cut into 3-in. strips
- 12 romaine lettuce leaves, thinly shredded
- 3/4 cup cilantro, chopped
- 3/4 cup Thai basil or sweet Italian basil, roughly chopped
- 12 oz. bean sprouts
- 24 rice paper wraps, about 8 1/2 in. in diameter

1. In a small bowl, whisk together creamy peanut butter, sesame seed oil, low-sodium soy sauce, ginger, hot sauce, hot water, rice vinegar, and sesame seeds. Set aside.
2. Spray a medium saucepan with cooking spray and heat over medium-high heat. Add extra-firm tofu and cook for about 2 to 3 minutes on each side until browned. Remove from heat and slice into 2-inch-long slivers. Set aside.
3. In a medium bowl, mix carrots, cucumbers, and green onions. Set aside.
4. In another medium bowl, mix romaine lettuce, cilantro, and Thai basil. Set aside.

5. Line up lettuce mixture, cucumber-carrot mixture, tofu, bean sprouts, and peanut sauce, in that order. On one side, have a large bowl with hot water in it.
6. To assemble: Dip rice paper in water for 15 seconds (if you do it longer, the rice paper will disintegrate). Carefully lay out rice paper on a flat surface. In center of rice paper, place $\frac{1}{4}$ cup lettuce mixture, $\frac{1}{4}$ cup cucumber-carrot mixture, $\frac{1}{2}$ ounce tofu strips, $\frac{1}{2}$ bean sprouts, and $\frac{1}{2}$ tablespoon peanut sauce. Fold over top, then fold in each side and roll again. Place seam side down. Serve immediately.

HEALTHFUL LIVING

The peanut is technically not a nut, but a legume, which means it's part of the bean family. It is high in protein and fat; is an excellent source of niacin; and is a good source of vitamin E, fiber, magnesium, and folate.

Black Bean Burgers with Sweet Potato Coleslaw

These spicy black bean burgers get even better when they sit overnight. Top them with creamy sweet potato coleslaw for a cool contrast.

Yield:	Prep time:	Cook time:	Serving size:
4 burgers with 1 cup coleslaw	20 minutes, plus 1 hour in the refrigerator	8 minutes	1 burger with $\frac{1}{4}$ cup coleslaw
Each serving has:			
531 calories	3 g fat	1 g saturated fat	0 mg cholesterol
19 g fiber	583 mg sodium		

1 tsp. corn or canola oil

2 garlic cloves, minced

$\frac{1}{3}$ cup green onions, chopped

$\frac{1}{4}$ cup red bell pepper, finely chopped

$1\frac{1}{2}$ cups cooked black beans (15-oz. can), drained and rinsed

1 TB. cilantro, chopped

$\frac{1}{2}$ tsp. cumin

$\frac{1}{2}$ tsp. chipotle chile powder

$\frac{1}{2}$ tsp. sea salt

Freshly ground black pepper

$\frac{1}{2}$ tsp. ground oregano

3 TB. nonfat plain Greek-style yogurt

$\frac{1}{2}$ tsp. lime zest

1 TB. lime juice

1 TB. egg white

$\frac{1}{4}$ cup cornmeal

$2\frac{1}{2}$ cups shredded cabbage

1 cup shredded peeled sweet potato (about 3 oz.)

1 TB. apple cider vinegar

1 TB. red onion, chopped

$\frac{1}{2}$ TB. honey

1 TB. cilantro, chopped

$\frac{1}{4}$ tsp. garlic powder

$\frac{1}{4}$ tsp. hot sauce (optional)

4 (4-in.) pitas

1. Heat corn oil in large sauté pan over high heat, then add garlic, green onions, and red bell pepper. Sauté 2 or 3 minutes until just beginning to turn brown.
2. Transfer to a food processor. Add cooked black beans and cilantro. Pulse until chunky but not a paste, about 3 times. Beans should be broken but still in small chunks. Transfer to a large bowl and mix in cumin, chipotle chile powder, $\frac{1}{4}$ teaspoon sea salt, black pepper, oregano, 1 tablespoon nonfat Greek-style yogurt, lime zest, lime juice, egg white, and cornmeal.

3. Form into four patties, place on a plate, and refrigerate for 30 minutes or up to 4 hours before sautéing.
4. While black beans are resting in the refrigerator, make coleslaw. In a large bowl, mix cabbage, sweet potato, remaining $\frac{1}{4}$ teaspoon sea salt, apple cider vinegar, red onion, pepper, remaining 2 tablespoons nonfat Greek-style yogurt, honey, cilantro, garlic powder, and hot sauce (if using). Toss to blend. Set aside in the refrigerator.
5. Heat a medium sauté pan over low heat. Spray with cooking spray. Add black bean burgers and cook about 2 to 3 minutes on each side.
6. To serve, place 1 burger on each pita and top with $\frac{1}{4}$ cup coleslaw.

HEALTHFUL LIVING

Over the years, beans have risen in nutritional and culinary status. Today in your average supermarket, you can find about 15 varieties of canned and 20 dried. You'll also find hundreds of varieties online.

Italian Polenta with Wild Mushrooms

Creamy Italian *polenta* is topped with a sauce of four different types of mushrooms: cremini, shiitake, oyster, and portabello. If you can't find them all, you can use white mushrooms with any other type.

Yield:	**Prep time:**	**Cook time:**	**Serving size:**
3 cups polenta and 2 cups mushrooms	15 minutes	35 minutes	3/4 cup polenta and 1/2 cup mushrooms
Each serving has:			
262 calories	8 g fat	1.5 g saturated fat	2 mg cholesterol
5 g fiber	316 mg sodium		

4 1/2 cups water
1 cup cornmeal
1/2 tsp. kosher salt
Pinch black pepper
1 TB. plus 2 tsp. olive oil
1/3 cup nonfat plain Greek-style yogurt
1 TB. plus 2 tsp. grated Parmesan cheese
2 garlic cloves, minced
1/4 cup red onion, chopped
1/2 cup sliced cremini mushrooms
1/2 cup shiitake mushrooms
1/2 cup oyster mushrooms
1/2 cup portabello mushrooms
1/4 cup white wine
1/2 cup crushed tomatoes
2 TB. fresh Italian parsley, chopped
1 TB. fresh oregano

1. Bring 4 cups water to a boil in a 3-quart pot. Slowly pour in cornmeal in a steady stream, over medium-high heat, for 1 minute while whisking. Decrease the heat to a simmer and cook, stirring occasionally, for about 35 minutes. About 5 minutes before it's done, mix in kosher salt, black pepper, 1 tablespoon olive oil, nonfat Greek-style yogurt, and 1 tablespoon Parmesan cheese. Cook for about 5 minutes more.
2. While polenta is cooking, set a large sauté pan over medium heat. Heat remaining 2 teaspoons olive oil. When hot, add garlic and red onion, and cook for 30 seconds. Stir in cremini mushrooms, shiitake mushrooms, oyster mushrooms, and portabello mushrooms. Cook until soft (about 5 minutes), then pour in white wine, crushed tomatoes, and remaining 1/2 cup water. Simmer 2 minutes. Stir in Italian parsley and oregano.

3. To serve, place $\frac{3}{4}$ cup soft polenta in a bowl, top with $\frac{1}{2}$ cup wild mushrooms, and sprinkle with remaining 1 teaspoon Parmesan cheese.

DEFINITION

Polenta is an Italian word for a thick mush of ground cornmeal boiled in water. In this country, it refers to both the dish and the cornmeal it's made from. Here it can be prepared soft and creamy or firm and dry (able to slice and fry), depending on what you're using it for.

Chapter 21

Delicious Desserts

In This Chapter

- Let fruit satisfy your sweet tooth
- Creamy confections to make your mouth water
- Sensational chocolate desserts

Just because you're on the TLC diet doesn't mean you have to give up dessert. You may, however, have to look at this part of the meal with a new attitude. Sweet treats are exactly that, a "treat" to be enjoyed on special occasions or only once in a while.

For most of man's existence, "dessert" consisted of some kind of fruit, perhaps with some dairy like cheese or yogurt and a small amount of sugar or honey—healthful, good for you, and tasty. Not surprisingly, most of the desserts in this chapter center on fruit. Fruits are low in calories; are high in fiber, vitamins, and minerals; and, most of all, provide the sweetness we love. These desserts also go easy on added sugar and fat.

Weaning yourself from the mountains of cookies, cakes, and pastries so readily available in our culture isn't easy. It takes time, patience, and discipline. For some people, the desserts in this chapter can help them get over the hump of controlling their sweet tooth and satisfying their palate with less sugar. Others may have to eliminate desserts and sweets altogether for a few months so they can tame their sugar cravings. If the latter describes you, you'll want to skip this chapter. Once those cravings are under control, you can re-introduce yourself to less-sweet desserts and experiment with the recipes in this chapter.

In addition to fruit-centric specialties, there are creamy concoctions like TLC Chocolate Pudding, brownies and cookies, and even a shortbread biscuit. All have a healthy component—yogurt, soy, whole grains, even beans—and all taste rich and indulgent.

Most can do double duty, such as the Caramelized Apples and Raisins, which also makes a great pancake topping, and the Roasted Peaches with Almond Oatmeal Crumb, also a perfect foil for low-fat regular or frozen yogurt. The fruits can be mixed and matched in any number of combinations, too, depending on the season—for example, you might use pears in place of apples, or raspberries in place of blueberries.

While fresh fruits are ideal, they aren't always available or accessible. In that case, frozen fruits are the next best thing, particularly for berries. Canned fruits are also a good idea and have a long shelf life. Be sure to buy less-sweet varieties packed in their own juice or in natural fruit juice.

The key to eating dessert comes down to one simple tenet: don't eat too much. If it's a more healthful dessert like the ones in this chapter, enjoy the serving size recommended; fit it into your daily or weekly calorie allotment. If it's an indulgent sweet that's not on the TLC diet, follow the one-bite principle. Take one bite, eat it slowly to savor the taste, and don't eat any more. You can save the remainder, share it, freeze it, or throw it out. Enjoy what you've eaten—usually that's all you need to feel satisfied—and move on.

Roasted Peaches with Almond-Oatmeal Crumb

Peaches roasted with a hint of maple syrup and then topped with an almond–oatmeal–graham cracker crumb are sweet and crunchy. This pairs well with creamy yogurt.

Yield:	**Prep time:**	**Cook time:**	**Serving size:**
$3\frac{3}{4}$ cups	10 minutes	25 minutes	$\frac{3}{4}$ cup
Each serving has:			
173 calories	5 g fat	.4 g saturated fat	0 mg cholesterol
4 g fiber	35 mg sodium		

8 to 10 small peaches, peeled, pitted, and chopped into $\frac{1}{2}$-in. pieces (about 4 cups)

1 tsp. vanilla extract

2 TB. maple syrup

$\frac{1}{2}$ tsp. cinnamon

8 low-fat cinnamon graham crackers, crushed (about 2 full sheets)

$\frac{1}{3}$ cup old-fashioned oats

1 TB. almonds, chopped

1 TB. corn or canola oil

1. Heat the oven to 325°F.
2. In a small bowl, mix peaches, vanilla extract, maple syrup, and cinnamon. Set aside.
3. Mix crushed low-fat graham crackers with old-fashioned oats, almonds, and corn oil until well blended.
4. Pour peach mixture into a $1\frac{1}{2}$-quart casserole dish sprayed with cooking spray. Top with graham cracker mixture. Bake for 25 minutes until bubbly and brown.

HEART-SMART HABITS

One ounce of almonds has 35 percent of the daily value for vitamin E and 8 percent daily value for calcium.

TLC Chocolate Pudding

Tofu gives this pudding its creamy consistency, while cocoa makes it rich and chocolate-y. Crushed chocolate graham crackers offer a slightly sweet crunch.

Yield:	**Prep time:**	**Cook time:**	**Serving size:**
2 cups	5 minutes	5 minutes, plus 2 hours chill time	½ cup
Each serving has:			
139 calories	4 g fat	1 g saturated fat	0 mg cholesterol
2 g fiber	59 mg sodium		

- 1 (14-oz.) pkg. soft tofu, drained, pressed, and patted dry with a paper towel
- 2 TB. water
- ¼ cup lightly packed brown sugar
- 2 pkt. stevia
- ¼ cup unsweetened cocoa powder
- 2 tsp. vanilla extract
- ½ tsp. instant coffee granules (optional)
- 8 chocolate graham crackers (about 2 full sheets), crushed

1. Gently pat tofu with paper towels to get rid of excess water. Set aside.
2. In a small saucepan, heat water, brown sugar, stevia, unsweetened cocoa powder, vanilla extract, and instant coffee granules (if using) until heated through and dissolved, about 3 minutes. Cool 5 minutes.
3. Place soft tofu in a food processor and slowly pour in chocolate syrup mixture while blending. Blend for 3 minutes, scraping down sides occasionally.
4. Pour pudding into a bowl. Gently fold crushed chocolate graham crackers into pudding. Divide evenly among four glass cups. Chill for 2 hours or overnight.

HEART-SMART HABITS

Experiment with different brands of tofu to find one you like. Some brands have more water in them than others. For this chocolate pudding recipe, try to buy a less watery type (like Mori-Nu brand).

Blueberries Topped with Lemon Ricotta Cream

Ricotta and yogurt blended with a touch of honey and flaxseed give this cream body and sweetness, while the tart lemon is a perfect contrast to the sweet blueberries.

Yield:	**Prep time:**	**Serving size:**	
2 cups	10 minutes	1 cup	
Each serving has:			
191 calories	6 g fat	3 g saturated fat	19 mg cholesterol
3 g fiber	100 mg sodium		

½ cup low-fat ricotta cheese

½ cup nonfat plain Greek-style yogurt

1 tsp. lemon zest

2 tsp. honey

2 tsp. ground flaxseeds

1 cup blueberries

1. In a food processor, place low-fat ricotta cheese, nonfat Greek-style yogurt, lemon zest, honey, and flaxseeds. Process for about 30 seconds to 1 minute until smooth and incorporated.
2. To serve, layer cream and blueberries in two small parfait glasses.

Variation: You can use practically any fruit for this dessert. Try this recipe with strawberries, raspberries, blackberries, or a combination of different berries.

HEART-SMART HABITS

To reduce the amount of saturated fat, you can use nonfat ricotta cheese in place of the low-fat cheese. The only difference is that the texture will be a bit drier.

No-Bake Peanut Butter Oatmeal Cookies

Make a big batch of these cookies and store them in the freezer. You'll need just one of these sweet, chewy, nutty cookies to feel satisfied.

Yield:	**Prep time:**	**Serving size:**	
18 cookies	20 minutes	1 cookie	
Each serving has:			
85 calories	4 g fat	1 g saturated fat	0 mg cholesterol
1 g fiber	2 mg sodium		

$\frac{1}{2}$ cup all-natural unsalted creamy peanut butter (see sidebar)

1 cup old-fashioned oats

$\frac{1}{4}$ cup ground flaxseeds

1 tsp. vanilla extract

2 TB. honey

2 TB. light brown sugar

$\frac{1}{4}$ cup dried cherries, finely chopped

1. In a medium bowl, place creamy peanut butter, old-fashioned oats, flaxseeds, vanilla extract, honey, light brown sugar, and cherries, and mix by hand with a wooden spoon until mixture begins to stick together.
2. Scoop by 1 tablespoon amounts, roll into a ball, and press down to shape into a cookie about $\frac{1}{2}$ inches thick. Place on a cookie sheet lined with wax paper. Chill in the refrigerator for an hour before serving, or place in the freezer for storage.

Variation: Replace the peanut butter with almond butter and the dried cherries with about 1 ounce shaved dark chocolate (72 percent). You can also add the chocolate along with the cherries, but you'll bump up the calories.

GOTCHA!

Beware of commercial brands of peanut butter that do not state that they're all-natural and unsalted. Many have partially hydrogenated fat (it keeps the peanut butter from separating) and salt added to the peanuts. In addition to being less healthful for you, this type of peanut butter will not work with this recipe.

Black Bean Brownies

Your friends and family will never guess that black beans are the secret ingredient to keeping these chocolaty brownies moist, low in fat, and rich tasting.

Yield:	**Prep time:**	**Cook time:**	**Serving size:**
12 brownies	5 minutes	25 minutes	1 brownie
Each serving has:			
145 calories	7 g fat	1.4 g saturated fat	0 mg cholesterol
2 g fiber	92 mg sodium		

1 cup cooked black beans, drained and rinsed

3 TB. corn or canola oil

½ cup egg substitute (equivalent to 2 egg whites)

¼ cup unsweetened cocoa powder

½ cup unsweetened applesauce

½ cup dark brown sugar

1 tsp. instant coffee granules

1 tsp. vanilla extract

¼ cup white whole-wheat flour plus extra for dusting

½ tsp. baking powder

¼ tsp. sea salt

¼ cup semisweet mini chocolate chips

3 TB. chopped walnuts

1. Heat the oven to 350°F.
2. Spray an 8×8 baking pan with cooking spray and dust with flour. Set aside.
3. In a food processor, place cooked black beans and corn oil and purée about 1 minute. Add egg substitute, unsweetened cocoa powder, unsweetened applesauce, dark brown sugar, instant coffee, and vanilla extract. Blend until smooth, about 30 to 40 seconds.
4. In a large bowl, whisk together white whole-wheat flour, baking powder, sea salt, and semisweet chocolate chips. Mix in black bean mixture and blend until incorporated. Pour into the prepared pan and sprinkle with walnuts. Bake 25 minutes. Let cool 15 minutes before removing from the pan. Cut into 12 pieces and serve.

Caramelized Apples and Raisins

Tart Granny Smith apples are caramelized with raisins and maple syrup on top of the stove in this simple dessert, which brings sautéed apples to a whole new level.

Yield:	**Prep time:**	**Cook time:**	**Serving size:**
3½ cups	10 minutes	5 minutes	½ cup
Each serving has:			
83 calories	2 g fat	0 g saturated fat	0 mg cholesterol
1.3 g fiber	2 mg sodium		

4 large Granny Smith apples, peeled, cored, and sliced (about 2 lb.)

2 TB. maple syrup

4 tsp. brown sugar

¼ cup loosely packed raisins

½ tsp. cinnamon

Pinch nutmeg

2 TB. chopped toasted walnuts (see sidebar)

1. Heat a large nonstick sauté pan over medium heat. Add Granny Smith apples, maple syrup, brown sugar, raisins, cinnamon, and nutmeg. Stir to coat apples.
2. Cook for about 4 minutes. Set aside and sprinkle with walnuts. Serve this fruit by itself as a sweet dessert or as a topping for pancakes, yogurt, or oatmeal.

Variation: You can replace the apples with pears and the walnuts with pecans. You can also change the spice to cardamom or ginger.

HEART-SMART HABITS

To toast walnuts, place nuts in a single layer on a baking sheet in a 350°F oven. Bake 8 to 10 minutes, checking frequently. Be sure to keep an eye on them—nuts can burn quickly. You can also do this in a hot, dry sauté pan over medium-high heat, stirring frequently for about 5 minutes.

Whole-Grain Crepes with Blackberry Compote

This nutty whole-grain crepe is light and airy and takes only minutes to make. Wait until blackberry season so you can find big, juicy berries.

Yield:	Prep time:	Cook time:	Serving size:
9 crepes	10 minutes	10 minutes	1 crepe filled with $\frac{1}{2}$ cup berries and 3 tablespoons sauce
Each serving has:			
153 calories	3 g fat	.3 g saturated fat	1 mg cholesterol
5 g fiber	61 mg sodium		

$1\frac{1}{2}$ cups water

$\frac{1}{2}$ cup freshly squeezed orange juice

6 TB. honey

$\frac{1}{2}$ tsp. cinnamon

$\frac{1}{2}$ tsp. cardamom (optional)

2 tsp. orange zest

4 tsp. cornstarch

$4\frac{1}{2}$ cups blackberries

$\frac{1}{4}$ cup egg substitute

$\frac{1}{8}$ tsp. sea salt

$\frac{2}{3}$ cup white whole-wheat flour

$\frac{1}{3}$ cup almond flour

1 cup low-fat milk

Nonfat yogurt for garnish

1. In a medium saucepan over medium-high heat, bring 1 cup water and orange juice to a boil. Add honey, cinnamon, cardamom (if using), and orange zest. Reduce heat to simmer.
2. Dissolve cornstarch in remaining $\frac{1}{2}$ cup water in a small bowl. Add to the saucepan. Bring to a boil, stirring constantly. Simmer 1 to 2 minutes until cornstarch becomes clear. Gently fold syrup into blackberries in a separate bowl. Set aside.
3. While blackberries are resting in syrup, make crepes. In a medium bowl, whisk egg substitute and sea salt until frothy. Slowly mix in white whole-wheat flour, almond flour, and low-fat milk (alternate while mixing).

4. Heat a nonstick 8-inch pan to medium-low heat. Spray with cooking spray. Pour $\frac{1}{4}$ cup crepe batter in the pan, tilting the pan to spread out batter over the entire pan. Let cook about 20 to 30 seconds, until edges start to curl. Flip over. Crepe will be slightly brown. Let cook another 10 to 20 seconds until lightly brown. Slide off the pan onto a flat plate. Repeat with rest of batter.
5. To assemble, place $\frac{1}{2}$ cup blackberry mixture in center of crepe. Fold end over and roll up. Serve with a dollop of nonfat yogurt.

Banana Pecan Maple Parfait

This Southern specialty dessert yogurt is sweetened with cooked sweet potato, then sprinkled with sliced banana and maple pecans. It's great when you have leftover sweet potatoes.

Yield: 4 parfaits	**Prep time:** 10 minutes	**Cook time:** 10 minutes	**Serving size:** 1 parfait
Each serving has:			
209 calories	6 g fat	.6 g saturated fat	0 mg cholesterol
4 g fiber	41 mg sodium		

1 large sweet potato, peeled and diced into 1-in. pieces

1 cup nonfat plain Greek-style yogurt

4 TB. pecans, chopped

4 tsp. maple syrup

2 bananas, sliced

1. Place sweet potatoes in a small saucepan over medium-high heat, with enough water just to cover. Cover and cook about 10 minutes until sweet potatoes are soft. Drain and rinse under cold water.
2. Once cool, mash sweet potatoes with nonfat Greek-style yogurt, or purée in a food processor for about 10 to 20 seconds until blended.
3. In a small bowl, mix pecans with maple syrup.
4. To assemble, layer $\frac{1}{4}$ cup sweet potato yogurt, $\frac{1}{4}$ banana, and $\frac{1}{2}$ tablespoon maple pecans in parfait glasses.

HEALTHFUL LIVING

In America, *parfait* means a layered dessert, usually with ice cream, cream or custard, nuts, syrup, and fruit. In France, however, *parfait* is a more general term and can be sweet or savory.

TLC Strawberry Shortcake

Freezing soft margarine is the secret behind making these low-fat, slightly sweet biscuits light and flaky. Topped with sweetened strawberries, this dessert is sublime!

Yield:	**Prep time:**	**Cook time:**	**Serving size:**
12 biscuits	10 minutes, plus 1 hour or more freezing time	12 minutes	1 strawberry shortcake biscuit
Each serving has:			
171 calories	4 g fat	.7 g saturated fat	0 mg cholesterol
3 g fiber	324 mg sodium		

4 TB. soft tub margarine
6 cups sliced strawberries
4 tsp. brown sugar
2 TB. water
1 cup white whole-wheat flour
1⅓ cups all-purpose flour
½ tsp. sea salt
1 TB. baking powder
½ tsp. baking soda
3 TB. honey
1 cup low-fat buttermilk
Nonfat yogurt for garnish

1. Place margarine in a small bowl and freeze for 1 to 4 hours (or overnight).
2. Place sliced strawberries in a bowl with brown sugar and water. Gently mix and let sit while you make biscuits.
3. Preheat the oven to 400°F. In a large bowl, whisk together white whole-wheat flour, all-purpose flour, sea salt, baking powder, and baking soda. Cut in frozen margarine until it is in small pieces. Working quickly, add honey and low-fat buttermilk, and using a wooden spoon, combine until mixture is just moist and will hold together.
4. Turn out onto a floured board and knead for about 15 seconds; dough will be slightly sticky. Roll out into a square about ½ inch in thickness, and cut straight down with a 2-inch round biscuit cutter. Make 12 biscuits (2 to 2½ inches). You may need to reassemble the scraps to make the last few.
5. Place biscuits on a stone or baking sheet lined with parchment paper. Let rest for 5 minutes. Bake in the oven for 10 to 12 minutes until lightly browned and risen. Cool.
6. To assemble, cut biscuit in half while still warm and fill with ½ cup sliced strawberries and juice. Top with a dollop of nonfat yogurt.

Appendix A

Glossary

aerobic exercise Any exercise that uses large muscle groups and can be maintained continuously (usually rhythmic in nature), like biking, walking, running, dancing, and skating.

alpha-linolenic acid (ALA) A type of omega-3 fatty acid (polyunsaturated fat) found only in plant foods, like vegetable oils, seeds, and nuts. In the body, it is partially converted to EPA and DHA, so you would have to eat a lot more to get the same amount of EPA and DHA in fish.

arugula A spicy, peppery salad green that is part of the mustard family and is high in vitamins A and K.

basal metabolic rate (BMR) The rate at which you burn energy, known as calories, while completely at rest. This includes all your vital bodily functions.

belly fat Excess weight around the abdomen. You don't have to be overweight to have belly fat. Abdominal fat is also called visceral fat because it surrounds your vital organs.

bisphenol A (BPA) A compound used in plastics, inside cans, on cash register receipts, and in hundreds of other things. In the body, it disrupts hormones and is particularly harmful for pregnant women and young children.

blood pressure The amount of force or pressure the blood exerts as it passes through the blood vessels.

body mass index (BMI) A calculation of height and weight used to determine whether a person is overweight. The drawback is that it does not take into consideration body composition.

bulgur Bulgur is a whole-wheat grain that is steamed or parboiled, dried, and then crushed or ground. It is a staple in Middle Eastern cuisine because it is an inexpensive source of low-fat protein.

caffeine A stimulant found in coffee, chocolate, tea, and cola products. Caffeine revs up metabolism, boosting energy and alertness. Too much can cause heart palpitations, shakiness, jitters, and sleeplessness.

cannellini beans Often called white kidney beans because they are large, with a kidney-bean shape, and creamy inside. They have a mild taste and thin skin.

capers The young flower buds of a caper plant that are pickled and cured in salt or a salt-vinegar solution.

caramelization This happens when sugar is heated to a high temperature; the heat causes the sugar to break down and produces a brown color and caramel flavor.

cardiovascular disease Any disease or condition that affects the function and structure of the heart. Coronary heart disease and coronary artery disease are both types of cardiovascular disease.

cholesterol An essential nutrient found in every cell in the body. Cholesterol is found only in animals and animal products, including fish. Too much cholesterol in the blood increases your risk of heart disease.

complex carbohydrates Starchy or high-fiber foods like 100 percent whole-grain bread, pasta, beans, whole grains, legumes, and most vegetables.

coronary artery disease A condition in which the arteries feeding the heart blood narrow, blocking blood flow to the heart and leading to tissue death or heart attack. Coronary artery disease is a type of cardiovascular disease.

coronary heart disease *See* coronary artery disease.

coping The thoughts and behavior you have in response to the perception of stress. Coping is done in an effort to lessen the negative effects of what's bothering you.

couscous A small wheat pasta that is available in two sizes: Moroccan couscous, or traditional couscous, which has tiny grains and cooks in five minutes; and Israeli couscous, which are larger round balls and served toasted.

cruciferous vegetables Vegetables that have a cross-shaped flower, found in the cabbage and mustard family. These include broccoli, cauliflower, kale, and arugula, to name a few. They are highly beneficial for good health.

curry powder A blend of spices, usually including cumin, coriander, red chilies, turmeric, and fenugreek. The mixture varies in strength and can be purchased mild or hot.

diastolic pressure Measures the pressure of your heart at rest (between heartbeats), when it is relaxed. It represents the bottom number of the blood pressure measurement. *See also* systolic pressure.

docosahexaenoic acid (DHA) A type of omega-3 polyunsaturated fatty acid that is found in fish and is good for the heart and the brain.

eicosapentaenoic acid (EPA) A type of omega-3 polyunsaturated fat found in fish that protects the heart.

emulsifier A substance that helps blend and stabilize a solution of oil- and water-based ingredients that would otherwise separate. Natural emulsifiers are egg yolks, peanuts, peanut butter, and cream.

energy-dense foods Foods that are high in calories but low in nutrient content. Soda and candy are very energy dense.

fiber Nonstarchy carbohydrate found only in plant foods, important for good health. Humans cannot digest fiber. Two types exist: soluble and insoluble.

grass-fed beef Cows that have been raised eating only grass found in pastures. Grass-fed cows are not given any grain products.

high blood pressure A blood pressure reading of 140 over 90 or greater. *Hypertension* is the medical term for high blood pressure.

high-density lipoprotein (HDL) A type of cholesterol that sweeps the "bad" LDL out of the bloodstream and keeps the blood clear. You want high levels of HDL, to reduce heart disease.

high-fructose corn syrup A highly processed sweetener extracted from corn and composed of a combination of fructose and glucose.

hummus A Middle Eastern dip or spread made from cooked chickpeas, sesame paste known as tahini, lemon juice, olive oil, and a few other spices.

hydrogenated or partially hydrogenated fats Man-made fats that are created by bombarding a liquid fat with hydrogen, turning the liquid fat into a solid.

impaired glucose tolerance (IGT) A condition that develops over time as a result of insulin resistance. It refers to changes in the receptors for insulin in your skeletal muscle and fat, leading them to become more scarce and less prone to allow insulin to bind to them. As a result, blood sugar stays high and there is increased risk of developing type 2 diabetes.

insoluble fiber Fiber that does not dissolve in water; insoluble fiber is important for digestion and is found in the cell walls and woody part of vegetables. It is prevalent in beans, whole grains, cabbage, and broccoli.

insulin A hormone secreted by the pancreas in response to high blood sugar levels. Insulin allows muscle and fat cells to use glucose (blood sugar) for energy and store as fat.

insulin resistance A condition in which cells have a lower response to insulin, meaning that it takes more insulin for cells to utilize glucose. Insulin resistance leads to excess abdominal fat, diabetes, metabolic syndrome, and other illnesses.

legumes A class of vegetables that includes beans, peas, lentils, and peanuts. These are high in protein and are a good source of vitamins and minerals.

lipid Fatlike substances that are found in the body.

low-density lipoprotein (LDL) A type of cholesterol that circulates in your blood. If it builds up, it sticks to your arteries and leads to coronary heart disease and heart attack.

metabolic syndrome A condition characterized by poor blood glucose regulation, hypertension, low HDL, high triglycerides and LDL, and abdominal obesity. It increases your risk for heart disease.

metabolism The sum total energy of all the chemical reactions that occur in your body.

monounsaturated fatty acids (MUFAs) A type of naturally occurring fat found in avocados, nuts, olives, and seeds.

muesli A type of grain mixture developed by a Swiss physician that usually includes oats, nuts, or seeds and dried fruit. It can be eaten plain or with milk.

National Cholesterol Education Program (NCEP) Part of the National Heart, Lung, and Blood Institute. The goal of the NCEP is to reduce heart disease in the general population by educating health professionals and consumers.

normal weight obesity A condition in which poor diet and a sedentary lifestyle lead to excess body fat around the belly, even in people who appear to be thin and maintain a healthy weight.

nutrient-dense foods Foods that are high in nutrients and low in calories. Most fruits and vegetables are nutrient dense.

obesity Having a body mass index (BMI) of over 30. *See also* body mass index (BMI).

omega-3 fat A type of unsaturated fat that's found in seafood and has protective effects on the heart.

overweight Having a body mass index (BMI) between 25 and 29. *See also* body mass index (BMI).

phytochemicals A broad array of beneficial nutrients found only in plants, important for good health.

pilaf Originated in the Middle East, but the standard way to cook whole grains in many Mediterranean and Latin countries, too. In a pilaf, the grain is sautéed or browned in butter or oil with vegetables for a few minutes before the liquid is added.

pita bread A traditional flatbread hailing from Middle Eastern and Mediterranean countries. It is often used to scoop dips such as hummus or to wrap falafel, and can be found in both white and whole-wheat forms in most grocery stores.

plant stanols and steroids Naturally occurring fatlike compounds found in small amounts in whole grains, vegetables, fruits, nuts, seeds, and legumes. In the body, these plant compounds block cholesterol from being absorbed.

plaque Thick, hard substance that builds up on your arteries. It reduces flexibility and narrows the arteries, causing blood pressure to increase and/or blocking the blood flow altogether.

poaching Gentle cooking method in which food is cooked in liquid heated to 160°F to 180°F, which means the water barely shows signs of bubbles.

polenta An Italian word for ground cornmeal boiled in water. Polenta can be soft and creamy or firm and dry (able to slice and fry).

polyunsaturated fatty acids (PUFAs) Fats naturally found in corn oil, safflower oil, soybean oil, and vegetable oil. Considered good fats when it comes to heart disease.

portion size The amount of food customarily consumed. Portion sizes have increased greatly over the years.

processed foods Foods that have been treated to change their physical, chemical, microbiological, or sensory properties.

protein Important nutrient your body needs to function. Proteins are composed of amino acids and are found in both plants and animals.

pulses A type of legume, pulses include lentils, dried peas, chickpeas, and dried beans.

quick-cooking oats Rolled oats that are flattened, making them thinner and faster to cook.

quinoa A whole grain originating in South America thousands of years ago. Quinoa is one of the few plant foods to contain all nine essential amino acids (proteins) the body needs. It is a small brown grain that turns translucent when cooked. It has a nutty taste and is excellent to use in place of rice.

refined carbohydrates Highly processed carbohydrates that have been stripped of their nutrient content or fiber to enhance shelf life or make them easier to eat or digest. Refined carbohydrates include white flour, white sugar, and white rice. Too much promotes belly fat.

refined sugars Sugars stripped of all nutrients during processing. White table sugar, cane sugar, and high-fructose corn syrup are refined sugars. Refined sugars promote belly fat.

risk factors Conditions or behaviors that increase your chances of getting a certain disease or condition such as heart disease or diabetes. Usually risk factors are seen in clusters.

risotto An Italian rice dish that uses a special type of round short- or medium-grain rice (usually Arborio rice) cooked in a broth until rich and creamy, often with cheese and butter.

rolled oats or old-fashioned oats Whole oat kernels that are steamed, flattened by rollers, and dried into flakes.

salt sensitivity A condition in which some people experience a rise in blood pressure directly from eating a load of sodium from food.

saturated fats Types of fat found only in animal foods like meat, dairy, fish, and eggs. Saturated fat contributes to heart disease, belly fat, and other illnesses. It's solid at room temperature.

serving size The amount of a single serving of food, based on a typical portion and determined by the USDA.

simple sugars Single- or double-bond sugars (monosaccharide or disaccharides) that the body readily absorbs. Glucose, fructose, and galactose are examples of simple sugars. Candy, soft drinks, and table sugar are examples of simple sugars.

soba noodle A Japanese noodle made from buckwheat flour. It has a strong, nutty flavor.

sodium An essential mineral that regulates blood volume and keeps the acid-base balance in blood in check. It is a main component of salt.

solid fats and added sugars (SoFAS) Solid fats are solid at room temperature; added sugars are put in during processing, such as when manufacturing sodas. You should reduce SoFAS to decrease your risk of heart disease.

soluble fiber Dissolves in water and is found in fruits, vegetables, beans/legumes, and oats. Soluble fiber is found in pectin and guar gum.

steel-cut oats Whole oat kernels (known as oat groats) that have been cut into small pieces by a steel blade.

stress Any threat to a person's physical or mental well-being.

systolic pressure The amount of pressure the heart needs to pump the blood out of it. This is the top number and generally is a higher number than diastolic blood pressure. *See also* diastolic pressure.

tahini Sesame seed paste, commonly added to chickpeas in hummus.

tapenade A condiment or spread usually consisting of puréed olives, capers, and anchovies.

teff An ancient grain that originated in Ethiopia. It is a tiny brown grain that is the main ingredient of injera, a spongy Ethiopian bread.

TLC diet Therapeutic Lifestyle Changes diet. The TLC diet is a sound approach to diet designed to reduce high cholesterol levels and decrease your risk of heart disease.

tofu A mildly flavored food made from pressed soybeans and formed into a smooth curd. It comes in three types—soft, regular, and extra firm—and easily takes on flavors.

trans fats Fats created by hydrogenating or partially hydrogenating fats. In the body, trans fats promote belly fat, heart disease, and other chronic illness, and are more dangerous than saturated fats.

triglycerides A form of lipid in the body that, in high levels, can increase your risk of disease. This can be caused by high sugar intake, high carbohydrate intake, and/or high fat intake.

type 1 diabetes A condition in which the pancreas is unable to produce insulin, resulting in cells that cannot take up glucose. It leads to high blood sugar levels, fatigue, malnutrition, and other conditions. If left untreated, it can be fatal.

type 2 diabetes A condition that occurs gradually, with cells becoming less responsive to insulin and resulting in higher blood sugar levels and the body's inability to handle carbohydrates. Type 2 diabetes can usually be controlled by diet and exercise, whereas type 1 diabetes requires daily insulin injections.

Type A personality A type of high-stress personality that is competitive, achievement-focused, and work-oriented. Can be at increased risk for health problems.

yogurt A type of fermented milk that originated in Turkey more than a thousand years ago. True yogurt contains probiotics, or good bacteria that can help promote a healthy digestive track and even boost your immune system.

Appendix

B

Resources

If you would like to learn more about heart disease, nutrition, and diet, the books, magazines, and online resources in this appendix are a great place to start.

Nutrition/Diet Books

Bloom, Jonathan. *American Wasteland.* Philadelphia, PA: Da Capo Press, 2010. Explains why and how America throws away nearly half its food.

Byrd-Bredbenner, Carol, Gail Moe, et. al. *Wardlaw's Perspectives in Nutrition, 9th Edition.* New York: McGraw-Hill, 2013. This basic textbook covers the principles of nutrition.

Kessler, David. *The End of Overeating.* New York: Rodale Press, 2009. Discusses how to take control of your eating from the perspective of brain function and behavior, based on a reward system.

National Heart, Lung, and Blood Institute, U.S. Department of Health and Human Services. *Your Guide to Lowering Your Cholesterol with TLC.* December 2005. Provides a good overview of the TLC diet.

Tessmer, Kimberly A., RD, LD, and Chef Stephanie Green. *The Complete Idiot's Guide to the Mediterranean Diet.* Indianapolis, IN: Alpha Books, 2010. Explores the basics of the Mediterranean diet and includes many simple-to-prepare recipes and meal plans.

Warshaw, Hope. *Eat Out, Eat Right*, 3rd Edition. Chicago: Surrey Books, 2008. This is a comprehensive guide to more healthful restaurant eating.

Welland, Diane. *The Complete Idiot's Guide to Eating Clean.* Indianapolis, IN: Alpha Books, 2009. Learn how to ditch processed foods and create amazing dishes using whole, all-natural foods. This book shows readers how easy it is to change their eating habits one step at a time, without breaking their budgets or sacrificing taste.

———. *The Complete Idiot's Guide to Eating Local.* Indianapolis, IN: Alpha Books, 2011. Everything you ever wanted to know about eating local—including what is local, why to go local, where to find local foods, and how to live a local lifestyle.

Wheeler, Claire, MD, and Diane Welland, MS, RD. *The Complete Idiot's Guide to Belly Fat Weight Loss.* Indianapolis, IN: Alpha Books, 2012. Diet and lifestyle plan for losing belly fat—includes info on diet, stress management, and exercise.

Whitney, Eleanor, and Sharon Rolfes. *Understanding Nutrition, 12th Edition.* Belmont, CA: Wadsworth Thomson Learning, 2011. This basic nutrition textbook tells you everything you need to know about fats, carbohydrates, protein, vitamins, and minerals throughout the lifecycle.

Culinary References

Asbell, Robin. *The Big Vegan.* New York: Chronicle Books, 2011. A cookbook with more than 350 no-meat and no-dairy recipes.

Bennion, Marion, and Barbara Scheule. *Introductory Foods, 13th Edition.* Upper Saddle River, NJ: Prentice Hall, 2009. This book explains basic food principles from a food science perspective, giving you the why as well as the how to make sauces, muffins, breads, and more. Great for beginners.

Dragonwagon, Crescent. *Bean by Bean.* New York: Workman Publishing Company, 2011. A bean cookbook containing more than 175 recipes for fresh beans, dried beans, cool beans, and more.

Joachim, David. *The Food Substitutions Bible, 2nd Edition.* Toronto, Ontario: Robert Rose, Inc., 2010. Detailed reference book on how to make substitutions in the kitchen.

Labensky, Sarah R., Priscilla R. Martel, and Alan M. Hause. *On Cooking: A Textbook of Culinary Fundamentals, 5th Edition.* Upper Saddle River, NJ: Prentice Hall, 2010. This comprehensive guide explores cooking ingredients, method, history, equipment, tools, and science. There's even a chapter on healthful cooking.

Natkin, Michael. *Herbivoracious.* Boston, MA: Harvard Common Press, 2012. Contain 150 vegetarian recipes; a great reference guide.

Speck, Maria. *Ancient Grains for Modern Meals.* New York: Ten Speed Press, 2010. Includes a wealth of Mediterranean whole-grain recipes for barley, farro, kamut, polenta, wheat berries, and more.

Newsletters and Magazines

Cooking Light
www.cookinglight.com
This magazine offers a compilation of healthy, great-tasting recipes in a consumer-friendly format. Every recipe has a photo.

Eating Well
www.eatingwell.com
This magazine is similar to *Cooking Light*, but more nutrition-oriented.

Environmental Nutrition
www.environmentalnutrition.com
The Newsletter of Food, Nutrition, and Health provides a good overview of new research in nutrition and other hot topics.

Harvard Health Letter
www.health.harvard.edu
This health newsletter from Harvard Medical School offers insights into nutrition science and health.

Nutrition Action HealthLetter
www.cspinet.org
Published by the Center for Science in the Public Interest, this newsletter offers nutrition articles, recipes, and news on the latest nutrition science.

Tufts University Health & Nutrition Letter
www.tuftshealthletter.com
This newsletter presents the latest nutrition research in short, consumer-friendly articles.

Online Health and Nutrition Information Sites

American Heart Association (AHA)
www.americanheart.org
National health organization devoted to reducing cardiovascular disease.

Food Marketing Institute
www.Fmi.org
The voice of food retail, mainly supermarkets.

Healthy Dining Finder
www.healthydiningfinder.com
Supplies nutrition information and helps you locate restaurants offering healthful items.

Livestrong
www.livestrong.com
Nutrition, diet, and health articles.

Mayo Clinic
www.mayoclinic.com
Health information provided by doctors, scientists, dietitians, and health practitioners from the renowned Mayo Clinic in Rochester, Minnesota.

Medicinenet.com
www.medicinenet.com
Site designed to provide health and nutrition information for health professionals and medical doctors.

MyPlate
www.choosemyplate.gov
How to put the dietary guidelines into practice.

Oldways
www.oldwayspt.org
A nonprofit group dedicated to preserving the "old ways" of drinking, eating, serving, and enjoying food; a big promoter of the Mediterranean diet.

Sciencedaily
www.sciencedaily.com
Review of nutrition and diet studies in press release format.

USDA Dietary Guidelines
www.dietaryguidelines.gov
Government-endorsed nutrition recommendations for the general public, meant to offer guidance for choosing a healthy diet.

WebMD
www.webmd.com
One of the best sources of health information online, written by doctors, dietitians, journalists, and health professionals; articles are reviewed by a medical board.

Whole Grains Council
www.wholegrainscouncil.org
Promotes different types of whole grains and offers consumers information on recipes, health benefits, nutrition research, and events.

Index

A

B

C

D

E

F

G

H

I-J-K

N

O

P–Q

R

S

T

U-V

W-X-Y-Z